It Is on You to Own You

A JAMAICAN NURSE'S JOURNEY
FROM POVERTY TO PROSPERITY

DELPHA CLARKE

DCE
Delpha Clarke
Enterprises

It Is on You to Own You: A Jamaican nurse's journey from poverty to prosperity
© *2023 Delpha Clarke*

www.delphaclarke.com

Printed in the United States of America
10 9 8 7 6 5 4 3 2 1 DCE 23 24 25 26

Library of Congress Control Number 2022910419

ISBN Paperback 979-8-9862872-3-2
ISBN eBook 979 8 9862872 1 8

Editing by Oasheim Editing Services, LLC and Inksnatcher
Cover design by German Creative
Photos by Delpha Clarke

Disclaimer

I would like to thank the members of my family, friends, and others portrayed in this book for allowing me to tell this story about them. I recognize that their memories of the events described in this book are different from my own. They are each fine, decent, and hardworking people. The book was not intended to hurt any family member, bash a culture, or bash other persons mentioned between these covers. Both my publisher and I regret any unintentional harm resulting from the publishing and marketing of this book to anyone noted herein.

Table of Contents

Part Three

Health Care: Misguided Cultural Mindset.....................**117**

Part Four

Freedom: Improving the Mindset **139**

Glossary of Terms

Ackee: Red, pear-shaped tropical fruit with poisonous seeds.

ACS: Acute coronary syndrome.

Bush baths: A ritual bath of herbs used to dispel evil hexes and illnesses.

CDC: Centers for Disease Control.

Cerasse tea: A bitter herb that purifies the blood.

Coal kiln: This is where wood is piled with a space left in the middle to light the fire. The result is charcoal.

Colporteur: A seller of religious books and tracks.

CNA: Certified nursing assistant.

COVID-19: Coronavirus pandemic.

CT: Computer tomography.

CTA: Computed tomography angiography.

CVA: Cerebrovascular accident.

Farm working: The United States created a program that recruited workers for farms and hospitality. In the early days it was farmwork only, and even though the program has since expanded to include other jobs and countries, we referred to it as farmwork (jis.gov.jm).

FAST: Focused Assessment with Sonography for Trauma. This is a focused exam used to identify fluid in the intraperitoneal (body cavity) or pericardial area (around the heart) in trauma patients.

Behaved ghetto: Gang street fighting.

Hopscotch: A playground game where you throw a small object (known as a lagger, but we called it a "man" in Jamaica) in the drawn rectangular boxes in a specific order. The person then hops or jumps through the different boxes without falling. If you fall, you lose. The number of players for this game is countless.

IV: Intravenous—in the vein.

Ludo: A table game with four players. A pair of dice is needed, along with each player having four "men," to travel around the board to what we call "heaven."

Macka tree: Also known as macka, this is a tree with pin-like thorns that can puncture your skin. Never try to climb a macka tree.

Marbles: A game in which a marble is placed between the thumb and second finger in the shooting position to hit other marbles out of a circle marked on the ground.

NCLEX: National Council Licensure Examination.

Number 11 mango: A sweet and juicy fruit. It is said that the mango received its name because it was coming from Africa on the slave ship and was found in the number 11 box, hence the name "number 11 mango."

Ockro: A flowering plant in the mallow family valued for its edible, green seed pods.

Patois: Spelled patwah locally, this is the dialect of the local people in Ja-maica. It's a mixture of the African tongue and English that was spoken to confuse the white man on the plantation, especially when the slaves were planning rebellion.

PCI: Percutaneous coronary interventions.

Medication pyxis: Automated medication dispensing system.

PPE: Personal protective equipment.

Repass: A gathering of friends and family, who offer food as a condo-lence and comfort when a loved one has passed away. A recollection of memories is shared about the one who has passed.

RN: Registered nurse.

RT: Respiratory therapist.

Saying: "One pussy kill cocky" means it is understood that one Jamaican man cannot have one woman but typically has many.

SDA: Seventh Day Adventist church.

Six form: The equivalent of twelve grades.

STEMI: ST segment elevation myocardial infarction—a heart attack. STEMI holds the highest mortality rate among all forms of acute coronary syndrome (ACS).

Stucky: A circle is formed, and the winning side after the toss-up goes in the ring. Each member takes turns and runs out of the circle while their opponents try to touch them. If they are touched, they cannot move unless another player from their side touches them. Then they are unstuck, hence the name Stucky.

SVT: Supraventricular tachycardia.

Tachycardia: Fast heartbeat, usually over 100 beats per minute.

Tachypnea: Rapid respiration over twenty breaths per minute.

Usain Bolt: A retired Jamaican sprinter.

Worms grumbling in my belly: Stomach growling due to hunger.

Yam head: Jamaican yam is a vegetable that is cultivated and consumed for its tasty and nutritious root tuber.

Zinc fence: Galvanized zinc used as property dividers.

I dedicate this book to my family.
May we never forget where we come from as we
look forward to building a stronger, more united future.

Introduction

From birth, man bears the weight of gravity on his shoulders.
He is bolted to earth, but man only has to sink below the surface,
and he is free.

~ Cousteau

ello, I am Delpha Clarke. I am a nurse, I am an author, I am an entrepreneur, I am a mother, I am a sister, I am a friend. I started writing because I was angry. Angry at getting a divorce, angry at allowing myself to be used, angry for not loving me for me. Through the cathartic process of writing, the anger has transitioned and transformed to where I now love myself and live for me and no one else. The writing through my anger resulted in this memoir about my life where, when I looked back, I could finally see the value of where I was born to where I am today.

My native language is Patois. The Jamaicans spell it patwah, just how it sounds. I interviewed a few of my family members and friends to add perspective to the Jamaican culture as I see it. Some speak with a mixture of English and Patois. I've added the English translation in brackets beside the words to make it easier for you to read and enjoy the story. Have fun with your new language, and when you visit Jamaica, be sure to practice some of your new words.

I love being a Jamaican. We have a special way of speaking about those we honor with pride. For example, we refer to our children as "my son," "my daughter," "my sister," no matter who we talk with. We are proud to identify our connection with each other and say that we love whomever we are referring to. You are not just a friend; you are *my* friend.

Sadly, for the longest time, I did not love my dark complexion, but I love it now. How dare I not? I love the fact that I am now a strong, independent Black woman. I would not ask for another skin color because I respect who I am and am proud of my history. No matter what color a person is, where they live, or what job description they have, it's important to be able to say this; I am proud of who I am.

As a nurse, I may be accomplished and capable and educated, yet I still often encounter and face racism in the emergency room from patients, peers, and staff. It doesn't surprise me anymore but it does bother me. It is not my mindset to look for it, and it is not my mindset to be offended; but as a Black woman, it is my mindset to talk about it openly and honestly, and to show others—both generations behind me and in front of me—that they do not have to allow it to impact who they are or who they become.

The racism is something to resist, confront, and deal with, but this can never hold me back. It is as important to me as my fight against poverty and a dysfunctional cultural mindset. If I can help others be victorious over poverty, racism, or anything that could damage their self-esteem, telling my journey will make them stronger.

My personality is strong, and the more I am pushed into a corner, the stronger and more resilient I become. I took the negatives along the way and made them my pillow at night. Getting a good night's rest has empowered me for the battles. However, I realize that not everyone feels that confidence and resilience, and I worry for the young women or men who have to face such adversity without a resilient mindset. I wrote this book to empower them, and to strengthen their resolve and confidence about facing these obstacles.

The truth is, we will all face racism and adversity in life, and it may come at the most unexpected times. We may be celebrating a win when it comes, delivered by a colleague or so-called friend and become de-flated at the events that occur. We must prepare our hearts and mind in advance, so that we cannot be defeated mentally or emotionally.

When I was growing up, times were hard. There was physical dan-ger everywhere.

The streets where I was born were covered with exposed and dangerous electrical wires, ready to strike if I took a wrong step. Life has been the same. I've learned some painful and valuable lessons from many missteps. I now choose my steps wisely and savor the power of celebrating a reward. I invite you to do the same. I would love for you to see how it is possible to accomplish great things when you choose better for yourself.

I have a bachelor's in nursing. Who gave it to me? No one else—, I accomplished it through many difficult steps.

I wrote my first book—this one—after years of thinking about it. What drove me to do so? *Anger* that transformed into a love for me, a desire to help others, and a passion for writing. I developed a heart for receiving help from professionals, sought guidance along the way from teachers and coaches, and remained committed to this task. I wrote this book not only for me but also for readers, and within these pages, I hope they will experience affirmation, empowerment, and even rest and growth.

In it, I hope you will see my deeply ingrained passion to help others.

I want to be exceptional in the things I put my fingers on because I am driven to be a better individual and to give of my best, and I hope to leave a positive impact on others.

I have goals. I have plans to reach those goals, and with my determination, I will work on my plans. I am fueled by my dreams, even if I'm not sure how to achieve them.

What is your struggle? I'd like to challenge you to look first at your surroundings and *examine* your mindset. You may be struggling through a challenge like a career change, a divorce or a lack of forgiveness for your parents. I hope by reading this book it will inspire your heart to be open to forgiveness, or maybe to love and appreciate someone, or perhaps to love yourself a little bit more. I hope that this book empowers you to live a better life that's free from anger and hopelessness, and that it reignites your commitment to you!

Perhaps you'll gain a new love for your husband, who you take for granted, or that friend you walked on yesterday, or the family member you stopped loving years ago.

I invite you to travel along with me through my life, and to experience for yourself a dose of inspiration to live your life better, create a new attitude, or learn something new about the Jamaica I know and love, and even the Jamaica I knew growing up.

If you think you are weak and cannot make it on your own, then that is true, but think again and learn to see that your strength lies within you.

Let go, be you, and enjoy the gift of freedom that comes from learning to love yourself.

I hope you enjoy my story.

Love,
Delpha

Part One

Poverty: Misguided Cultural Mindset

Chapter 1

A Typical Day

RADIO:

"GDM MEDICAL CENTER, THIS IS MEDIC ONE."

"GO AHEAD, MEDIC ONE."

"WE HAVE A SIXTY-EIGHT-YEAR-OLD FEMALE IN RE-SPIRATORY DISTRESS. DIAGNOSED WITH COVID-19 TWO DAYS AGO. OXYGEN SAT OF 80 PERCENT. ON 15 LITERS OXYGEN VIA REBREATHER. BLOOD PRESSURE 89 OVER 57, PULSE 130, TEMP 102. ETA 7 MINUTES."

"COPY, MEDIC ONE."

As I walk by the nurse's station, the charge nurse alerts me, "Delpha, you are getting a respiratory distress in Room 16. COVID positive. Sounds septic."

"Got it." As I attempt to get the crash cart, my mask, and other PPE readily available, I see the triage nurse with an EKG in hand.

"We have a possible STEMI (ST segment elevation myocardial infarction) in triage, Doc, and he does not look good," she says, handing the EKG to the physician. "He is complaining of central chest pain, radiating to his left shoulder. According to his wife, this started fifteen minutes prior to presentation. He is diaphoretic, cold, and clammy."

Leaning on the crash cart, I wait for the doctor to make the call. We only have Room 16 available for a critical patient, and by the sound of it, this is one.

"Yes, this is it. Let's fax to the cardiologist. Call a code STEMI," he says.

Vick, triage nurse: "Where do you want the STEMI?"

"Room 16. Let's clear 17 for the respiratory distress, guys. I will get the STEMI kit."

I grab the crash cart as curious onlookers—visitors with their relatives in the passage—look at everyone moving at an accelerated pace.

RADIO:
"CODE STEMI-ER. CODE STEMI-ER."

The triage nurse wheels the "patient-on-bed" into the room, and the defibrillator pads are on his bare chest while he clutches at them. As per the American Heart Association guidelines, any patient that needs percutaneous coronary intervention (PCI) should be treated within ninety minutes of arrival at the emergency department (ED). We call it "door to balloon time"—the time the patient arrives at the ED to the time he is in the cath lab getting reperfusion (restoration of blood flow) of his coronary arteries. The coronary arteries take blood to the heart muscles. When there is a blockage, as in the case of a STEMI, the patient starts to have chest pain with shortness of breath. This patient is having an anterior wall myocardial infarction (MI), in short, a heart attack. The worst kind of all.

"0-2 sat on monitor, 91 percent, BP 98 over 67," I say.

The respiratory therapist, Kevin, starts him on two liters of oxygen. His saturation needs to be at least 94 percent.

I grab supplies to start his intravenous access (IV) while Todd starts a second line.

"Is your husband allergic to any medication?"

The man's wife in the corner shakes her head no. I look in her eyes and see the fear there. Her life partner is in grave trouble.

"Administer heparin 5,000 units IV," says the physician.

The patient grabs my hand, "Don't let me die."

I look directly into his eyes and ask, "What's your name?"

Breathlessly he says, "John."

"We are doing everything we can, John."

The feeling of impending doom can be a sign of MI in these patients. *I am also getting a feeling of doom* while the team gives 100 percent to prevent this.

"Doc, are we giving any heparin infusion?"

"IR doc said to skip that part."

"Delpha, Cathy from IR is on the way."

"Okay. I am going down with John."

Usually the interventional radiologist nurse (IRN), an ER nurse, and a respiratory therapist, if needed, go with the patient. Today I have a feeling we will need Cathy.

"Heparin 5,000 units administered."

"Hi, Delpha, what's the story?"

"Hey, Cathy. This gentleman started having central chest pain radiating to left shoulder. Started thirty minutes ago while working in his backyard. His wife gave him four baby aspirins. He has bilateral IV access 18 gauge to the left basilic vein and 20 to the lower forearm. I gave him heparin 5,000 units. He has no allergies. Known to be hypertensive and hypercholesteremia but noncompliant with meds. We started him on two liters oxygen via nasal canula. He is pale and diaphoretic. We need to move."

"Cathy, what's his weight?"

"What's his weight, Jane."

"Ninety-seven kilograms."

"Jane, what time was the heparin given?" she asks, leafing through her sheet as she walks across the room toward us.

"08:45."

"Kevin, do we have enough oxygen in the tank to take him to IR?"

"We are a go, Delpha."

"Let's go, guys." Double-checking everything, we roll out with me pushing his bed.

"John, we are taking you to IR (interventional radiology) for reperfusion of your artery."

He gives a thumbs-up.

As we roll out of the ER with the team, the feeling of my patient dying hits me again. *Don't die, John, don't die on my watch.* I hate this feeling. *Is everybody where they need to be? Oh, I can feel it. Don't die, John.*

My eyes move from my patient to the monitor. I am super alert. I hear Cathy speaking in the distance to John's wife as we move at a fast pace. I look at Kevin with his ambu bag (a portable respiratory bag) in hand, ready if anything should go wrong.

> **RADIO:**
> **"SEPSIS ALERT. ER ROOM SEVENTEEN. SEPSIS ALERT.**
> **ER ROOM SEVENTEEN."**

"John, we are almost there. You're doing good." I try to ignore the announcement, knowing full well it is another patient I have to deal with. I know the work will be continued by another nurse. *I can only manage one patient at a time, one at a time!*

John raises his hand slightly but it falls limply on the bed.

"What's wrong?"

He starts to have gasping respirations. I stop pushing his bed while Kevin starts administering oxygen to him.

"John, John," I say as I simultaneously search for his carotid pulse. I feel nothing.

I press the button on my radio, looking directly at Cathy so she knows I will not be returning to the ER, "Code blue, code blue to IR!" I jump on the stretcher and start chest compressions, thirty compressions to two breaths.

"One, two, three … thirty …"

Kevin squeezes the ambu bag twice.

"COPY THAT, WILL ALERT IR," belts out of my radio.

Cathy continues to push me and the patient to the IR, me doing CPR and Kevin tagging along awkwardly with the ambu bag as I count.

"…twenty-eight, twenty-nine, thirty…"

Kevin knows what to do.

"Delpha, hang on. I gotta turn a corner."

I steady myself going through the doors of IR while continuing with the compressions. The IR team is already prepared for the patient.

"One, two, three …"

The IR nurse checks John for a pulse. "No pulse, continue CPR, flat line on the monitor."

She takes over the compressions … four, five …

I get off the stretcher and walk out as the IR team continues chest compressions on John. I hope he will make it.

An ER nurse must be proactive, stay physically fit, have grit, take the initiative that's within their scope, and move. Keep the tears at bay until they can curl up in bed at home, away from the drama, when no one is around.

"Delpha, Sandra is assisting you with the respiratory distress in Room 17," says the charge nurse as she acknowledges me with a gentle pat on the back and moves herself to assist another patient.

Great, I start the shift with a bang, and it will continue—these twelve hours will go rapidly.

I gear up in my PPEs to see Sandra staring at me through her eye shield. "Not only do you owe me a steak dinner but also coffee, Delpha."

"Nah, you deserve two steak dinners *plus* your morning coffee. Thanks for helping me."

I assess the patient and look at the monitor. I see her SAT (oxygen saturation) is still in the 80-percentile range, despite her 15 liters via the rebreather. Tachypneic at 32 (fast respiration, it shouldn't be over 20 breaths per minute), tachycardic at 126 (fast pulse). *Hmmm.*

"Hi, ma'am, what's your name?" I ask the patient.

She looks confused at my question. *I love my accent, but at times like this, not much.* On a regular day, in a regular situation some of my patients can't understand me. Now, with these masks, it is worse. I try to speak slowly and louder so she can understand me. I know my throat will be dry and sore later.

"What—is—your—name?"

"Kel—"

I touch her to reposition her oxygen probe and realize how cold and blue her fingers look.

"Hey, Sandra, we need respiratory. She needs BiPap, she needs ABG, EKG. Stat."

"Hey, speedy, relax! Respiratory was paged. Remember, Kevin went with you to IR (intervention radiology). He is the only RT today. His colleague called in sick. Doctor Skillet saw Kelly here and ordered all these things. He also called a sepsis alert on her," says Sandra.

"Okay, did we get blood work?" I attempt to listen to her airway with my stethoscope.

"Kelly here is a hard stick (hard to get a vein), but I was able to get one IV and sent the first set of cultures. I need a second line and a second set of cultures. EKG is done and shows sinus tachy (tachycardia). Doc ordered two liters of fluid. He went to put the other orders in," reports Sandra.

"I really owe you a *few* steak dinners," I say as I move toward the computer to check the other orders.

"Yes, you *do* owe me—I carried extra supplies in the room for the IV. It's on the counter, Delpha."

"Sandra, Doc ordered methylprednisolone, antibiotics, anxiolytic, and Remdesivir."

"I will grab the meds," Sandra says as she turns to head out.

"Okay, I will be the dirty nurse and you be the clean nurse, Sandra."

Whenever we are in a COVID room with a patient, the nurses have developed a system whereby whatever we need, someone on the outside will get it; hence the "clean and dirty nurse" phrase. This saves time and conserves supplies, so we don't have to change out of the PPE (personal protective equipment) so often. The drawback to this is that you are hot and thirsty, and the possibility of passing out from dehydration and exhaustion grows. It's a miserable state and high risk for a frontline professional.

Luckily, I am able to get a second line on Kelly and a second set of cultures.

"Kelly, I have two sets of antibiotics for you and your remdesivir. Your white blood cell count came back elevated, meaning that there is an infection going on. I also have your antiviral meds. That is for the COVID-19."

She shakes her head to indicate she understood as she struggles to breathe, but she is tired from her struggle, and I fear she might go into respiratory arrest. *Where is that BiPap, Kevin? Hurry, come on.*

I start her antibiotics when Kevin enters the room with the BiPap machine. *Yesssss, sweet, he is here!* "Hey, Kevin, thanks. Just in time. Here you go."

Kevin goes to the opposite side of the bed so I can administer the meds through the IV. "Delpha, here we go again."

"Indeed, we do." I touch Kelly's shoulder. "Kelly, the calvary is here, yeah." I smile at her even though she can't see it, but she can hear the joy in my voice. *Never show anxiety to the patients when you are in fighting mode to save them. This makes them panic and makes* the situation *worse.* I continue to smile in my voice.

"Hi, Miss Kelly, I'm Kevin, your respiratory therapist. I will be placing the machine on you to help your breathing. It will be a bit uncomfortable, but it will help."

My patient nods affirmatively again. Kevin takes a blood sample for her ABG (arterial blood gas). Leaving the room, he says, "Delpha will be back in a few minutes to let you know the results."

"Cool, thanks, Kevin."

Kelly's skin is pale, and her lips appear blue. I know she is a smoker with COPD. *Still not out of danger. Hang on, Kelly.*

"How are you doing now, Kelly?"

She looks up with her mask on and nods, indicating that it's better.

I stay with her, administer her meds, and ensure everything was started before I leave the room. I check the monitor again—*SAT 91 percent, BP 110 over 60, pulse 120, and respiratory rate 28*—okay, this is a little bit better.

"Okay, Kelly, I will check on you very soon. Just relax and breathe, okay?"

"Can I have some water, please?"

"When I return, I will give you ice chips."

"Thanks."

My radio squawks as I peel PPE off in the room and discard it, feeling a lot more comfortable now that she is on the BiPap machine.

> **RADIO:**
> **"DELPHA, YOU HAVE A NEW PATIENT IN ROOM 19."**

Well, this is a typical Monday indeed. They are always the worst in my ER. I head toward the bathroom before going to see my new patient and answer a text from Nathaniel.

> **"MOM, WHEN ARE YOU COMING HOME?"**
> **"HI, MY SON, I WILL PICK YOU UP AT 7:45 P.M. LOVE YOU. LATER."**

I enter my new patient's room and say hello. "My name is Delpha, and I will be your nurse for today. What's your name?"

"I am Nicholas James, but you can call me Nicky."

I smile at that because I have a nephew with the same name, and we call him Nicky as well.

"My doctor sent me to get a blood transfusion. My hemoglobin is 6.5."

I sit on the chair and listen to my patient as he gives an account of his reason for coming to the ER. After he completes his story, I think, *At least I get one easy case. Blood transfusion and possible admission. Case closed.*

I smile to myself only to be greeted with hyperactivity outside. *What now?*

"Delpha!" shouts my charge nurse again. *I guess I will know soon enough.*

"Do you have a Trauma Nursing Core Course certificate (TNCC)?"

"Yes."

Can you assist the trauma that's coming in? ETA about five minutes now. We will be getting one critically ill patient and we may need to Medi Vac him to a trauma center. The first one coming in has abdominal trauma. You can work with Sandra in Room 1; she will brief you. The others can be saturated between fast track and sub-acute. I called for additional hands, and I have alerted the OR (operating room).

Oh boy. I peep in on my COVID patient, Kelly.

"Hey, Delpha, the ABG (arterial blood gas) came back showing respiratory and metabolic acidosis. Going to increase her oxygen so she can breathe off some of that CO_2."

"Good plan, Kevin. Can you give her a few ice chips as well while you are in there?" I say as I hurry down the corridor to Room 1.

As I enter the room, I see Sandra, who came to my rescue earlier, getting her room ready, along with Todd our medic. It's now my time to return the favor.

"Delpha, do you want to write?"

"Why not? A change in role will do me good."

Todd and I will do all the work while you scribe. Todd, you down with that?"

"Let's do it, Sandra."

"Yeah, we got this."

"Any more info on what's coming in?" Doc asks as he enters the room.

"Yes, Doctor Skills. We have a twenty-one-year-old guy, uh, unrestrained driver, sounds unstable. BP 81 over 46, pulse 118, SATS of 95 percent on room air. Obvious bruising to chest and right upper abdomen. He is in a collar and on a backboard. They started him on normal saline."

"Okay, he has a narrow pulse pressure and abdominal bruising to the right upper quadrant. This could possibly be liver laceration leading to hemorrhagic shock. I have already asked the surgeon to sit in on this with us. Todd, if we do not have two lines, place a second one. Have the OR team prep."

"Vick informed the OR already."

"Good. Do we have everything we need in the room ready?"

"Yeah, we are ready, Doc, Sandra said she's double checking everything."

"He may not be stable enough for transfer. Let's get the FAST done and see."

"Why did they not transfer him to a trauma center?"

"Good question, Delpha; they have no immediate available transfer. We need to stabilize or go directly to the OR. Luckily Doctor Phills, our surgeon, has a background in trauma."

If our patient responds to fluid and stabilizes, we can hold off on surgery and do a CTA (seeing any blockages, aneurysms, or leaks in arteries by injecting contrast into the blood vessels) of the abdomen and pelvis. *This patient is a priority. All others can wait.* I glove up.

"Paramedics are here," Todd alerts us.

"This is Patrick, a twenty-one-year-old restrained driver who drove over a dead body in the road. Lost control of the vehicle and went into the guardrail. He was going at approximately 75 mph."

Oh God, I have a lot of questions but no time for that now.

"Currently complaining of pain and swelling to right upper quadrant of abdomen. Noticeable bruising seen. Blood pressure also noted to be falling. The lowest we got was 77 over 44. This improved to 82 over 40 after one liter of fluid. Pulse 136. He is now lethargic and diaphoretic (increased perspiration). Patient transferred to trauma bed."

The trauma doc begins the primary survey. He goes through it rapidly.

"Patrick, do you know where you are?"

"Hmmm," Patrick groans.

RECORD NOTATION:
PATIENT CLOTHING CUT AND REMOVED, THROWN IN A CORNER OF THE ROOM. MONITOR ATTACHED, SAME SHOWED SATS OF 94% ON ROOM AIR, PULSE OF 123, BP 86/35.

"I need the ultrasound machine."

"Right behind you, Doc."

"Second IV in. Eighteen gauge to the left AC (antecubital)."

"Hey, he's got fluid in his intraperitoneal cavity. He needs surgery stat! Give him another liter while enroute to the OR."

As I grab my radio to let Vick know, I hope that Patrick will make it. This is someone's son, someone's brother, someone's friend.

A minute later, Sandra and Todd rush out of the room to the OR.

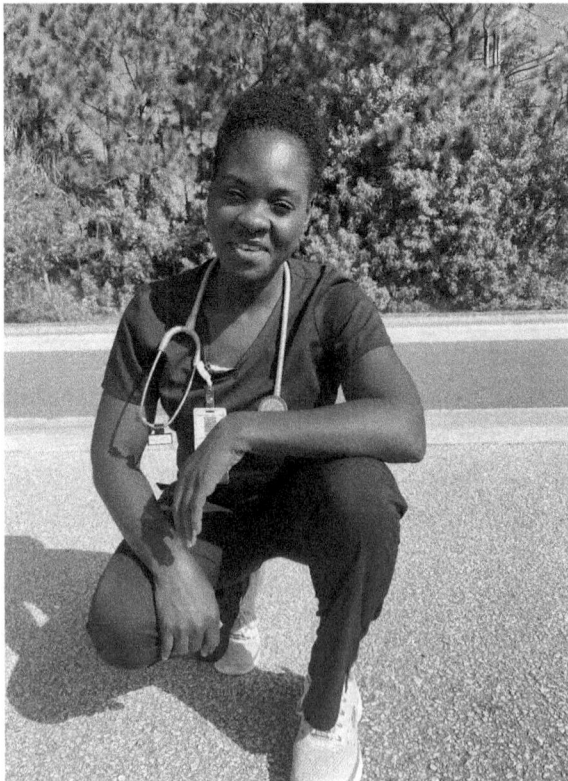

Image 1: Delpha.

Chapter 2

Time to Take a Breath

I sat in my car in the parking lot after work that evening before I drove home to pick up my son, Nathaniel, and I was too tired to even sanitize my shoes. I started to think about how fragile life is.

Today was a mess. Not all my patients will get the chance to feel the morning sun on their faces ever again. John was only fifty-nine-years old. He was not ready to die. He said, "Don't let me die." Did I do enough for him?

There is pain in the air. His wife was devastated when I went to the cath lab to drop off a more stable patient.

I have never gotten used to the sadness of it in my eighteen-plus years of nursing. And I don't know these people but for a short time in my life. The few hours I've spent with them may seem like a short time, but those hours are huge because I give them 200 percent of me to save their lives and when they die, it hurts.

Thankfully, Carol had her family and friends around to support her. She hugged me and thanked me for giving my best, but I did not feel deserving of those words because her husband did not make it.

I wonder if Patrick will make it. He is only twenty-one years old. He has to; it's not his time yet. Am I questioning you, God, when I make such statements? I don't know. Patrick had a laparotomy done and was now admitted to the ICU. *Yes, he may totally recover physically, but will he fully recover emotionally after such a trauma?*

The happier side of today was that Kelly turned around and could even tell Kevin not to call her "Miss" as that made her feel old. This we smiled about. At least one positive outcome! I have seen so many patients die during the COVID-19 pandemic so that news was amazing.

Today I had one COVID patient to take care of, but I can remember having four patients at a time. I had to continue to change in and out of my PPE gear, going from room to room and being both the clean and dirty nurse. Sometimes I would go in the room and forget something. Then I had to change all over again. There was no one I could call to give a helping hand. Nurses were sick from the virus or simply exhausted.

We were just too short-staffed. Doctors were also putting new orders in as the lab results came through. If I were a Duracell® battery, I would have shut down. The cycle repeated itself as my patients were admitted and a new set arrived. I was thirsty, I was tired, I was stressed, I was going through a divorce, and it was just God alone that took me through that period. *Thank you, God.*

It was scary for us in the beginning, when not even the CDC was sure how to approach these cases. For others, it brought home the awareness of the sudden closeness of death. So many were dying.

We who are living take such things as waking this morning for granted. We head straight on in the day without saying "God, thank you for another breath." I am also guilty of this.

We are nurses, we take care of others, and when we go home, we nurse our husbands and children. *Sandra had to leave in a hurry because her husband was involved in another car accident. I hope it's not too serious and he will be okay. She had tears in her eyes when she ran out of the ER.* The nurse's job is one that is

continuous. *I will check on her later after I get Nathaniel—my smarty-pants son. I check my watch.*
   Oh God, it's now 8:30. I need to brace myself for his reprimand. After all, I will be two hours late.

Frozen behind the steering wheel of my car, I craved this time to unwind.

Being a single parent is not an easy job. I was so angry at my ex-husband. Life is so short, yet he lived like he did not care. I hated feeling unloved and uncared for in my marriage. I felt like I was the only one fighting. I was the only one seeing into our future and making plans for those times. If couples value life, they will value each other. In these times, people think only of themselves, and that was our downfall.

   We were both nurses fighting to save others, yet we could not save our marriage. Jack refused to look and see that loved ones were losing each other. I was angry because he did not value the importance of what we shared. I was angry because I felt used and abused, betrayed, and trodden on. I am human. I deserve to be loved and cherished, not by any man but by my man. But he was too busy entertaining himself and others. He refused to fight for our growth and development. I guess he must have thought that I was not worth it. Things in life that we don't treasure, we lose.

   Many first responders suffered in silence during the pandemic. How do you heal through the constant trauma we all faced day after day?

   One person cannot build everything in a relationship. It's the little thoughtful moments that count. The moments when the love of your life pops in your head for no apparent reason, or the little big moments when you both sit and work out how the mortgage will be paid this month. These are the little big moments that count and make the union stronger.

I pulled the car out of the parking lot. *I could have had so much.*

It is so vital for you and your partner to work together. I never want to go back to poverty. That is why I worked so hard to provide a good life for Nathaniel and me. I was the healthy one in the relationship. He had a heart condition, and you would think he would have been smart about it. *My son could be home with one of us now instead of at a babysitter's house. I am mad at him, but this anger ...* I had to release it and so I wrote. It really helped me to gain a different perspective on things.

Being a nurse has its rewards and challenges. Sometimes I question myself to see if those challenges are not too much. Sometimes I do feel like it is more than I can take. *There was so much pain in the air today.* Parents came flying in wondering if their son or daughter was still alive. The fear in their eyes mixed with hope for good news. It is such a wonderful feeling when they ask about the most important person to them, and in that moment, you can smile and say they will be fine. The sudden relief in their eyes is priceless.

Therefore, I continued to be a nurse. Despite a shortage of colleagues to lighten the burden of the influx of patients, especially during a pandemic; despite management finding fault with the one mistake I might have made, or they think I did, compared to the 99 percent good that I did under stress, I continued to push on. *Despite shortage of equipment to make the job easier, I will push on. Despite being talked down to because of my color, I will push on. Any negatives anyone throws at me, I will push on.*

Sometimes we need to also remember to stop ourselves and be a human being. *I wear the nurse's hat, I wear the job of a sister, I wear the job of now a single mother whose child right now is upset with her*

"Hi, son." I waved goodbye to the sitter and mouthed thank you to her as I pulled out and headed to my final destination for the night.

"Mother, you are late."

"I know, I am sorry."

"You cannot have me staying here and there. I need to be in one place, and you need to stop being late. I have been waiting for you for hours."

"Okay, I will try my best. It's a pity, Nathaniel, that people don't put a time as when to be sick for my convenience and yours."

I looked at him through the mirror and saw how angry he was. It melts my heart when he is not happily doing something crazy and being a kid. My only child, my sunshine. If he only knew the day I'd had, he would have hugged me (after my shower, of course) and said, "Mom, I understand." But I leave the drama at work to face this drama at home. I try to separate them, but sometimes it's too hard.

Sometimes I wonder if Jack asks himself what he did wrong, or if he did anything at all to contribute to the success of our marriage. I also keep asking myself what I could have done better. *What about our son? Did he not care?* Sometimes I wonder if the path I have chosen is worth it—this divorce, working so hard to provide a different future for Nathaniel than what Jamaica might have offered him. If I had not taken this path, I often wonder where I would be—maybe still suffering in Jamaica. Scraping for food. What mother wants to see her child hungry?

"Okay, Nathaniel, we are home. I need to do my routine."

"Okay." He slammed the door to the car and raced into the house.

I changed my clothes in the garage before entering the house. I tossed them into the washing machine and got it going as I did not want to take any pathogens or germs home to Nathaniel. I quickly jumped in the shower and had a steam bath, letting it cleanse my lungs. *Ah, that feels so good. A nice cup of warm lemon and ginger tea will help keep my im-mune system strong. It sounds perfect about now.* I came out of the shower and went in search of my youngster.

"Can I get my hug, now that I am clean? Mama loves you always. I have your back. Never forget that."

"I know, Mom. Why can't you work somewhere else?"

"My job is hard, but I love it. This is what I want to do, Nathaniel. I cannot promise that I will never be late again, but I will try my best to leave a little earlier. Me coming late to pick you up does not mean that I don't love you because with all my heart, I do."

"I know you do, Mom. I just don't like staying with other people."

"I know—just bear with me until I figure it all out. In the mean-time, I will fix something yummy for dinner."

"Okay, Mom."

"In the morning, I will run with you to school. Your mama must keep healthy to keep up with her son and do her job effectively. I love you so much."

"I love you too, Mom."

As I sat and looked out at this beautiful view before me, I smiled because I knew life must get better.

My phone vibrated on the kitchen counter with a text message.

> DELPHA, MY HUSBAND IS IN THE ICU. HE WAS THE OTHER CRASH VICTIM MEDIVACKED TO THE OTHER HOSPITAL WHILE WE WORKED ON OUR CRASH VICTIMS IN THE ER. I WON'T BE IN TOMORROW. PRAY FOR US, PLEASE.

> OH MY, SANDRA, I AM SO SORRY TO HEAR THAT. I WILL KEEP YOU IN MY PRAYERS. CAN I DO ANYTHING FOR YOU? WHAT ABOUT THE KIDS?

> MY SISTER HAS THEM. WHEN THEY COULD NOT GET A HOLD OF ME, THEY CALLED HER. OH, DELPHA.

SAY NO MORE. IF YOU NEED ANYTHING, AND I MEAN ANYTHING, SANDRA, I AM HERE.

THANKS SO MUCH.

I WILL VISIT YOU GUYS TOMORROW. HANG IN THERE.

After this last text, I could not help but ponder life again. It is not easy walking this nursing path alone. Thank God for my relatives and friends. Thank God Sandra had her support system in place.

Chapter 3

Pondering Life

*T*he experiences one goes through in life might make us think that life can be limitless. I tend to have a greater appreciation for life after I have emerged from a dark place. I love the feeling of freedom and discoveries of my new potential that comes from my experiences.

When does it happen for you? When might you wake up and say, "Yes, this is it. It is time to shine, it is time to grow, it is time to leave the past behind." When do we let go of the past and keep it from spoiling our current state or our future? Let's look to the future and start to plan, dream, and just enjoy life. Will some of us ever get that opportunity? What will it take for us to wake up and decide to love and accept ourselves to be the stars we were born to be?

What experiences do we need to ascertain and realize how beautiful, strong, fearless, and independent we are? It took betrayal for me to realize that I deserved more than what I was getting from my (now ex-) husband at the time. That was when I said to myself, "Yes, this is me, and I should be living loved, shining, and growing, with him in my rearview mirror."

My realization occurred when the Jamaican sun came shining through with opportunities I could not see during my dark times. Being born into poverty, the oppression I had given permission to—out of ignorance to that poverty mindset—fed my low self-esteem. I realized it was time to open my eyes, choose courage to walk through the new door opening in front of me, let go of the grief, stop being so naive, dry my tears, and take action toward a better way of thinking. I wanted a better life.

Born in Jamaica, I am the twenty-second of twenty-three brothers and sisters—a huge family. I never was sure how I fit in until much later in life. I was sheltered and protected by my bigger brothers and sisters and sometimes even by the youngest, Marie. She is fierce; she knows what she wants and goes for it. She got married at the age of eighteen to the man she loved and left Jamaica for "the great big America." Initially, the family was against this marriage. She said, "Hell to all twenty-two of you," and went off to live her life. How dare we try to get in her way! Today, she is happy with her husband of twenty-four-plus years, and they are still in love. I wondered at times if I could ever be that fearless. I wanted to be like her when I grew up. I still admire her courage and continue to look up to her.

I am the only one who was not as street-smart as my siblings because the older ones looked out for me. I just loved books and they opened my mind up to other ways of thinking. I read a lot of fiction that developed my imagination. It was also a form of escape while I planned my flight out of poverty. I now understand that the reason for the life I have today is because I have taken responsibility for myself and own my better decisions.

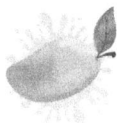

Power Thought

In hindsight, I see the value of being happy and living in the moment. I have learned to not wait for tomorrow to appreciate myself or to show appreciation to others. Fears can be killers of my dreams, and I want to overcome them by applying the "The 5 Second Rules," according to Mel Robbins in her book *The 5 Second Rule: Transform your Life, Work, and Confidence with Everyday Courage*. Robbins states that when we have the "do it now (in five seconds)" attitude, we don't spend time thinking too much. In turn, this prevents the what-ifs from setting in, and we start the action of taking control of our immediate situation and being the organizer of our life. Five-four-three-two-one—go for it. Do not think about it. Step out and fly.

As an adult, I will no longer wait on anyone to grant me permission or to agree with my thoughts. I no longer need anyone's approval like I did with my old, dysfunctional, cultural mindset. In fact, during the editing process of this book, my editor has given me the endearing pet name, "the Roadrunner." I know I am the person God created me to be as I continually change my life for the better today. I can now see his hands have always been there, even during the times I could not see them.

Thus, *It Is on You to Own You*—a book on how to cancel a misguided cultural mindset to loving who you are and find the person you are meant to be. It is my story of the courage and determination I chose to help me on my path to get where I am now. My hope is that it inspires you to make that first little change in your life and know that the possi-bilities for a better you are endless. I have learned to love who I am and will share how I came to find the person I was meant to be.

Chapter 4

Jamaican Roots

Living in a Culture I Knew Little About

The culture of Jamaican society is quite different from what tourists see when they come to visit. I was not privileged to experience this beauty growing up because we had no money to visit the tourist destinations on the island. When I left Jamaica, I experienced that Jamaica through the eyes of the tourists because I often heard comments that made me curious:

"Delpha, I love the beauty of your country."

"Delpha, I love the beaches of Ocho Rios."

"Delpha, I climbed the falls, and the water is so clean."

"Delpha, I love the food—the curried goat, the oxtail, ackee, and saltfish."

I knew about the food because once in a while, my mamma would cook these beautiful dishes, but I was not familiar with the classy side of the island. As a native, I only knew the real culture of Jamaica. Poverty. We didn't know any better because it was all we had, so we worked with the limitations of our resources. When I saw our differences with others who lived better than us, it gave me a new hunger for a better life. For example, I was never concerned about the secondhand clothes, the tight-fitting shoes, or the lack of school supplies. My friends at school shared their lunch from their lunch pans at school because I had none. I know hunger because I lived it. In the summer I would go with Judith and Suzan—my two elder sisters—and sell scrunchies and headbands on the street in downtown Kingston to have money to buy supplies for school.

Let me introduce you to my tribe. My father had many kids, of which he took responsibility, even for those who were not biologically his. When my mother and he met, she brought kids of her own into the relationship.

The cultural mindset in the 70s and 80s, especially in the poorer part of the country, was that the more kids you have, the more manly the community views you. Young men would taunt each other, pat one another on the back, and be congratulated for having many children. You were classified as a real man or as "having a strong back." When a young man did not have kids, he was considered weak, and no respect was given by his colleagues.

This way of thinking could possibly stem from the time of slavery, when the men were used as breeders on the plantations. The mentality passed from generation to generation. Once freed into a new way of living, they were on their own to build a roadmap to a new way of freedom thinking. It was on them to take responsibility for survival where they now owned their situation. Instead of "breeders," the people transitioned to a different type of survival with their kids, who were now the pension plan for their old age—when their backs could no longer meet their needs for survival. It was all they knew.

More than twenty years later, the cultural mindset is improving somewhat. Men are wising up and having fewer children. For the average family to truly give their children everything they need, it can be challenging. Can you imagine feeding such a tribe as ours by parents who earned below minimum wage, especially in Jamaica, a third world country? Think about it. How would you survive as a child or parent?

Genealogy Children for Thelma and Ivan Clarke and other parents				
Mother:	Father:	Birth Name	DOB	Pet names
Thelma	Ivan	Beverley	1959	Judith
Thelma	Ivan	Julian	1971	Suzan
Thelma	Ivan	Sonia	1973	Gina
Thelma	Ivan	Shelly	1975	Shelly
Thelma	Ivan	Delpha	1977	Sherene
Thelma	Ivan	Marie	1979	Bunza
Thelma	Donald James	Donovan	1967	Dingy
Thelma	Whittingham	Wayne	1963?	Wayne
Thelma	Ronald Richards	Paul Richards	1969	Taddy
Thelma	Lloyd Ricketts	Harold Ricketts	1961	Peter
Thelma	Lloyd Ricketts	Altimon Ricketts	(Died at six months old)	
Gwendolyn	Ivan	Verol	1954	Speedy
Gwendolyn	Ivan	Eric	1957	Littleman
Gwendolyn	Ivan	Veronica	1959	Lorna
Gwendolyn	Ivan	Keith	1960	Keith
Gwendolyn	Ivan	Angella	1963	Joy
Gwendolyn	Ivan	Vinora	1964	Novlett
Gwendolyn	Ivan	Michael	1965	Keble
Gwendolyn	Ivan	Andria	1966	Donna
Name Unk	Ivan	Jahleith	1954	
Name Unk	Ivan	Pauline	Deceased	
Name Unk	Ivan	Garfield	Deceased	
Kathrine	Ivan	Karen	1972	
Total: 23 children				

My mother is Thelma, married to my father, Ivan Clarke. They had six girls together. Mamma came to the relationship with five boys, although some had already left home. My father Ivan had eight children with Gwendolyn, who he had never married, and four children with four other mothers, who he had not married either. It's interesting to note how the birthdates of the siblings by different mothers overlapped during the same years.

The age difference from the youngest to the eldest did not allow for everyone to live under the same roof at one given time. I have sisters with age differences of more than twenty years. Many had already left home or were married with families of their own, making room for more children to arrive in the Clarke tribe. I recall that there were ten of us under one roof at one time.

Of my siblings, we have zero to four children each. Some are married whereas others are not. We have learned to not have as many because we do not want to repeat what happened to us. My dream was to have three boys and I am blessed with one son. Sometimes, caring for him is all I can handle as I have been diligent about shifting my poverty mindset to one of abundance.

We siblings all view one another as 100 percent blood sisters and brothers. We do not use the word "half." It is just not an acceptable term.

Can you imagine building sibling relationships with twenty-three people, much less all of the nieces and nephews? That is a huge tribe! Some of my siblings have passed away, and not all are close, but we try to stay connected from time to time. The six girls became closer because we lived in the same home and were closer in age. Mama liked to keep the kids together and Papa made sure no man came close to our inner circle. He protected the yard with dogs, and a brother or two were always close by.

The Jamaican old age pension program is a cultural mindset where the Caribbean men and women, and third world countries in general, are of the notion that the more kids you have, the better your pension. Parents ingrain in the brains of their children, "It is your responsibility to take care of me when I am old." I once heard Mama arguing with my neighbor, who, for some reason, mistakenly spoke badly about one of us children. Mama threw her hands in the air in anger, then placed her left hand akimbo and pointed the other one over the zinc fence as if the other party could see her, and said in our Jamaican Patois, "Lef mi pickney dem alone, dem a mi old age pension!"

She spun around and kicked off her slippers angrily at the door and stomped back into the house. This translates to "Leave my children alone, they are my old age pension!" She planned for us to take care of her: therefore, she did not want anyone to molest or harm her "insurance policy." The day will come when she can no longer take care of herself. My mother is eighty-one years old and receiving the benefits of her Jamaican old age pension as she is well taken care of by us, her children. She lives with Marie or myself and often travels to Jamaica to stay with my other sisters. Her pension "rotation" plan works quite well for her. The benefit for us is that our children have the opportunity to enjoy a relationship with her during her staycations.

Jamaican patois (Jamaicans spell it patwa) is the language used by the local people and a tradition for the uneducated. The famous Louise Bennett—a Jamaican poet, folklorist, and educator—states that we should be proud of this language. Patois is a mixture of French, Spanish,

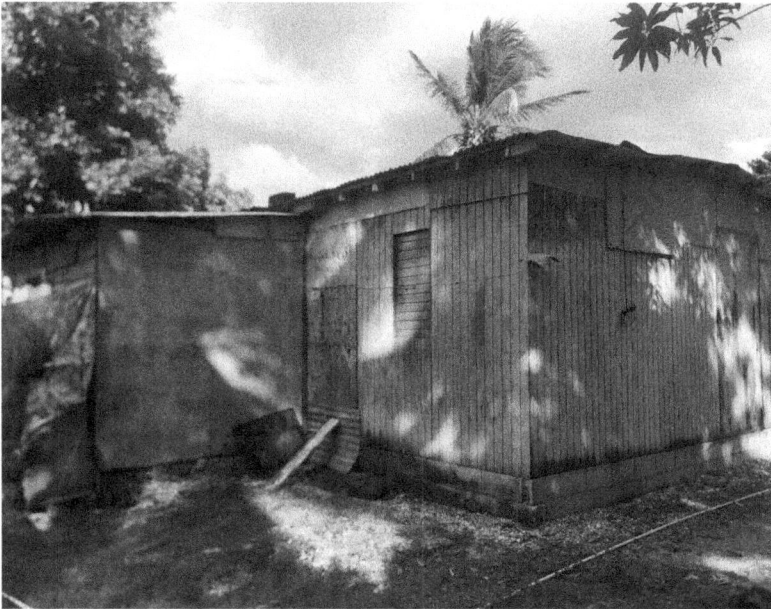

Image 2: House where I grew up in the community of Frazers Content also know as Redpond.

and English and is colored with the African tongue. It was developed in the 17th century. This dialect often allowed us to speak against the oppression from slavery as the White man could not understand the language. My mother's use of it against the neighbor shows how deeply ingrained this Jamaican pension plan was for her future.

Likewise, I must unlearn this type of pension plan as I am empowered by education to constantly learn new ways to improve my life. I want my child to build a future for himself without the pressure of supporting me as a parent. There are good things to say about both ways.

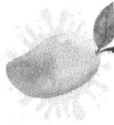

Power Thought

I am proud to be a Jamaican. It is who I am, my identity, for today, tomorrow, and forever, even though I am now an American citizen. I have fought the good fight to run from poverty. When I get depressed, regretful, or weary, I remember the days of hardship with my brothers and sisters. I don't want pity from anyone; I want education so that I can learn better ways to live life and impart to others. I am fiercely committed to pushing forward and I will not give up. I fight not only for myself but for them and my future generations.

To my fellow Jamaicans, embrace the patois, the mother tongue. Embrace the parts of you that make you Jamaican. It is part of us, and it contributes to our uniqueness as a people. We are a very creative people; we build the best. We share our time and little resources we have to help one another because we truly care. If the favor can be returned, it is good. If it can't be returned, all is still well. If you choose not to return the favor when you have the resources to help, it will hurt us, but we will move on. We expect our rewards to come from God. If we have to do it again, we will do it to a fault and sometimes to our own demise. We don't even want our enemies to suffer like we have suffered. For the most part, a Jamaican will help you. There are always exceptions anywhere.

I will forever celebrate this special part of my Jamaican soul.

I am further shedding this cultural mindset where twenty-three children are my old age pension and have embraced the abundance that one child brings. I can afford to clothe, educate, and feed him without anyone looking down on him, nor do I have to suffer the pain of seeing my child experience hunger, like my mother did with so many of us.

Chapter 5:

Elder Care Comparisons

I love the Jamaican idea of caring for family, but I want to do things differently so it is not so cumbersome or a strain on time. This helps us all relax and enjoy each day that comes as best as we can. There will be more time for meeting emotional needs instead of constantly worrying over duty or where to get the money. The retirement funds are an asset that will buy time, on which I place an extremly high value. I look forward to when not just me, but my family and friends also, can focus on our families without being encumbered by money.

I have worked to adjust my thinking as I embrace the American culture. I continue to save for retirement. My Jamaican roots are a blessing to my new American life because I now know what to avoid and know what I should do. When I arrived, I had no savings for retirement in this country. I look at my forty-plus years and wish I could have started saving for retirement from the day I was born. I have also looked at the fact that my son, Nathaniel, is now being cultured differently; he is more Americanized than Jamaicanized due to his exposure to the diversity his school has to offer. His education is very different from the one I received. Things have certainly changed.

When I am in my seventies and eighties, I want to continue to live in my own home. Ideally, this home will be located near a body of water, where I can see the sunshine forming diamonds as it glistens off the surface. The wind will dance on the water with a tension. The tension allows the birds in flight to glide along with the waves. I want to admire the view from my picture window, where I feel the wind as I speak this dream into existence. I feel the same freeness as the birds, and the breeze caresses my face with the curtain as I gaze into my future. To have the time to dream is a luxury. For me this is contentment, freedom, and peace.

I cannot and will not use the same phrase my mother used about her children being her old age pension. I choose to be responsible for myself and must put proactive plans in place so that my growing financial investment will do the work when my back can no longer support me. I choose to embrace this new concept of investing for my future.

I have learned that I do not need the permission of my family and am free to make choices for myself. In America, I more than likely will end up in a nursing home. This transition is an eye-opening thought. I now choose to learn everything I can about investing wisely with my finances.

In our Jamaican society, we do not believe in nursing homes. According to Denise Eldemire's study of the elderly population in Jamaica, she revealed that approximately 40 percent of the largest elderly population in Jamaica is receiving a government pension that is not sustainable to meet their basic needs. The burden is then left on the rest of the family. This is what third world and underdeveloped countries understand about getting old.

I do not want to be a burden to Nathaniel. I want to depart this world with a smile on my face, knowing that I have given my one son the gift of time and financial freedom from my care. I hope to be able to say that I lived above and beyond just an existence of survival. I want Nathan to be able to say that my legacy is that I planned well and lived a life of caring, giving, laughing, and loving. The only difference about my Jamaican soul is that I am becoming an educated Jamaican soul as I seek to learn to do things better. I want to impart this wisdom to my fellow Jamaicans who want something better for themselves too.

I learned that elder care is the opposite in America to what it is in Jamaica—the idea of you living with and taking care of your parents or other incapacitated family members is not totally embraced in the USA like it is in Jamaica. If I remain in America (a lot more about that later), the thought of how I might be cared for concerns me. I would love it if I could look forward to the hope of living with my children and not be a burden here in America. When I cared for my father in his last days, it was out of a sense of duty and love. Despite that, it dominated my thinking and my life as his care became more demanding. Our lives were so intertwined that when he passed away, I could not turn off my routine. I was accustomed to being with him. In hindsight, I loved to spend time with him and felt it gave me purpose. The deep concern was burdensome though. When I was not around, my mind would be on him. I worried his blood sugar might run low, but luckily, I was there to correct his hypoglycemia before it went too low and he passed out.

Once I was introduced to the concept in America about saving money for retirement, I could see that the gift of time in our lives is the most valuable asset to allow money to work for me. I want to give this gift of time to my next generation. I want Nathan to be free to expand his mind in his studies, to enjoy his childhood and not have to worry about hunger. I care for him now, and I plan for our future by saving money for my retirement care.

My father died at the age of seventy-five with the same Jamaican pension plan that his children would take care of him. He left nothing behind. There was no life insurance, no savings, no land, no education—meaning that he could not even read. He was very street-smart. He knew he had a lot of kids, so he leased a house with a lot of land space. He enclosed his property with a zinc fence (known in America as galvanized) for protection, to keep out unwanted neighbors who might want to steal what he planted in the garden.

My little yard was in the community of Frazer's Content and often called Red Pond. I don't know why it was called that considering there is no pond or anything red. You would first be greeted by our produce garden. Guava flooded the senses as you entered the gate. We would often climb the trees and swing from the guava tree's thick cream branches. These same branches would sometimes meet our bottoms when we misbehaved. Close to the guava tree was a small patch of sugar cane. Whenever we were hungry, we would all gather and cut cane to temporarily sooth the hunger pangs as we feasted, laughed, and played with each other. Dasheen grew out of our earth. We often dug it up to cook with cornmeal dumplings. Served with a bit of butter, the heat melted it to perfection. A mouthwatering bite tasted dry and sweet as we savored the flavor. Often, I did not wait long enough before my first bite to fill my belly. My impatience left my tongue and roof of my mouth sore from the burns.

Next to the dasheen patch, banana trees grew. The white yam grew up the bark of the ackee trees with its seed proudly displayed. The garden greenery was so abundant, we could sometimes hear the whistling sound of the wind passing through the plants from inside the house.

Other produce included pop choy (Americans call it bok choy), okra, sweet potatoes, breadfruit, and, of course, mangoes. This was the custom with the poorer families who had some land. Unbeknownst to us then, we were eating organic produce. It was the very best and it came from our garden. Papa often went to the local shop and put other food supplies on credit such as cornmeal, flour, butter, and sometimes chicken back, which was our main source of protein which is mostly fat and bones. At the end of the week, the shop gave him a bill that was crazy high. I guess interest would grow on this credit within a week. My mother did not like the idea of putting our food on credit, but what other choices did she have? It was either that or we could go hungry more often than usual.

I can remember sometimes our garden would be low on produce and we did not know where our next meal would come from. My sister Gina reminded me that when we were younger, I would go into the garden and pick the yam head (the seeds) from the vines of the tree. This was bitter when we cooked it, but we ate it anyway with whatever meat was available. My Jamaican soul certainly learned how to think outside the box for survival.

My mother went around doing what we call a day's work, which is washing people's clothes. She'd walk for miles to get to work and then back home to us five days each week. I can remember anticipating her return.

We had a big open field outside our zinc gate, which was called The Commons, where sometimes the green grass would meet us at the knees, so tall that it looked like waves in the wind, plus macka trees to climb in some areas. We'd stand to look and see when Mama might come because she often carried a bag full of mangoes home to us. We'd all run with bare feet, surrounding her and the bag as she set it down. We impatiently waited for permission to swoop down and grab a juicy mango. We called them "number 11" mangoes because it was said the box always had the number 11 labeled on it, coming from the African ship back in the days of slavery. I can still remember the sensations of eating the meaty, juicy, sweet number 11 Jamaican mangoes and feel the juice running down my face.

My father was a man of many talents. He worked on ships at the wharf in Jamaica. In his older years, he opened a shop where he did shoe repairs—we had dirt roads and a lot of foot walkers. He also sold ground provisions and charcoal; the coal kiln made the charcoal. In Jamaica, we call this the coal skil. Once you stopped by his shop, he would give you something to eat or give a talk while he repaired shoes. His favorite meal was the chicken back. Since it is all skin and bone, the skin produces a lot of oil, especially when fried, but my father knew how to cook it well. He often seasoned it with scallion, thyme, onions, and, of course, powdered seasoning from the local shop. I licked my fingers every time! Everyone loved it when he cooked chicken back.

I keep asking myself if my father was really smart. Did he not realize that having so many children was costly? Why could he not restrain himself from having so many women? We were experiencing hunger, we needed clothing and proper education. I know he saw this, yet he continued to live the way he did. His joy also came in the form of drinking, smoking, and playing dominoes with his friends. After all, this was all he knew. Common sense should have dictated to him that he needed to stop, but it appears that the only thing that could stop him was a bullet.

This bullet came in the form of a cerebrovascular accident (stroke). He could not read, but knowledge not only comes from reading, it also comes through the form of education from your own experience and taught by others. If my father was smart, then perhaps I would not be here and I would not have so many brothers and sisters. Yet, the positive effect is that I am not alone in this world. I meet patients every day who have no family and no one to support them, especially in their times of ill health. I don't want to know what that feels like without my tribe. In short, my father did what he knew. Because of this, I can only love him.

He was a people person, well respected by the community. He was given several pet names: Tawee or Wiggy, which had no specific meaning but showed how well-loved he was. He was known as the man with a lot of children, girls more than boys. My sister Lorna shared some history—someone once sent a man to kill my father. He might have messed with someone's woman, who knows? The name that man got was not a name that he was familiar with, but when he saw it was my father, the man showed him the gun.

"They sent me to kill you," he said, and turned and walked away. My father's loving nature to help those in need, whether by helping fix schoolchildren's shoes, providing a meal, helping to build a house, or digging a grave, meant you could always count on "Tawee." Maybe these names were given to him because of his kindness. This type of living was a daily lesson we took with us into adulthood.

My mother had the opportunity to leave us to go to the United States to work a housekeeping job in the hotel industry. We referred to this as farm work, officially called the US Farm Work Program, where one can get employment legally in the United States. Now, it is referred to as Overseas Employment in a variety of industries. She often said that she did not leave us before because she did not want us to be abused by a stepmother. My mother was so strict. The only time we had free rein was when we attended church all day on Saturdays. Sundays and Wednesdays were reserved for church in the evenings. We were not allowed to visit my uncle, who lived at the entrance of the lane close to us. We were only allowed to visit our friends who were Christian.

We were surrounded by rusted zinc fences, The Commons, and dirt roads with a lot of potholes. A lane was only wide enough for two people to walk side by side. Even though the streets I grew up on were not paved with gold, to say the least, our type of life made us strong and determined.

The only time my father flogged me with his belt was an unforgettable lashing, all because I went to my sister's house. We were not allowed to visit others, no one. Her husband was supposedly abusive. My mother often said, "I have a lot of you so you can all play with each other."

To this day, we are awfully close because we were each other's best friends. Mama made sure we grew together as brothers and sisters who looked out for each other, despite her having so many of us. She taught the bigger ones to take care of the younger ones, but sometimes us younger ones took care of the bigger ones. Life was good in this respect. I am not sure how my mother was able to teach all of us to become so street-smart, but she did. As I mentioned before, I am the only one who was not as street-smart because I read so much, and the older ones looked out for me.

Growing up, my parents' main concern was to make sure that we were fed to meet our all-consuming need for survival, like our African ancestors. Food and shelter were a higher priority to my father than learning to read and write. Once the survival mode was satisfied, we could move on and began to crave knowledge. Not all of us were able to fight our way out of poverty. Some lacked the know-how, and some could only see themselves in poverty. Some simply didn't want to know and preferred handouts. Some became lackadaisical and expected those who were doing better to give them a handout. We are a group who value family relationships and connections in our community. Because of this connection, we continue to feel for and give to one another, sometimes until it hurts the one giving.

The cultural assumption is that once one becomes more educated, which is one of the paths toward making more money, the demand from the community grows. The African mindset for generations has assumed that because of this, the one who has more should give to the one with a lesser income. Even the individual who has more tends to give because they feel inherently compelled to do so. We as a people need to understand that once the income improves for one, so will the standard of living. With this new standard of living, there are higher expenses. I know that even though my income has improved, I must still live below my means to set money aside and plan for my future. People tend to forget that everyone has expenses. The conflict lies between the disparity of the cultural mindset and my new abundance mindset. As I work to break free of the handout mindset to where I am today, taking responsibility for my needs, this change is the most important one I must accomplish to achieve success. True, I want to rescue everyone and feed the world. If I do that, it will break me. I must choose to make these difficult changes and work toward an easier life, plan for retirement, and be free. It is okay for me to live a little. I'm not rich. I still struggle because I have given too much, to where I do not have enough to meet my responsibilities. In order for me to have enough to support myself, I must stop giving too much. I want to have enough. My enough is not riches but enough to relax and not have to work so hard. Enough that my belly is full and that I never know hunger again.

I became an expatriate of Jamaica because I desired a more comfortable way to live once I knew it existed. I learned how education, any education, could improve my outlook. My confidence and thinking changed once I learned to read. One day I would like to return to my homeland, like many other Jamaicans I know, and be a teacher who inspire others to choose ways to improve their lives. I want to share the education I've obtained. Currently, expatriates are not able to do so because of the risks of being targeted, robbed, and possibly killed for the little they have worked so hard to achieve. I want something better for the people of my nation, but only if they want to learn. The question is if the Jamaican people want something better for themselves. Some may be content with life as it is.

There is nothing wrong with that if one is making an honest living. However, if this way of living is not acceptable to society, my hope is that my story will inspire my people to examine where they are and the endless possibilities that one can achieve from gaining new perspectives. For the African generation to grow financially wise, or let's just get a little closer to home—for Nathan to have a better life than me, I must first teach him about the financial world of the culture we now live in, how to handle money, and how to not just spend but save and give as well. He must learn the value of money by working for it. He's learning that he can receive an honest income in exchange for hard work. I find things for him to do that will encourage responsibility and educate him about business: capital, income, expenditure, decision-making, and negotiation. Better yet, he can learn the principle of money management and become an entrepreneur or a boss for a company, if he chooses. From the time he has learned that rewards come from putting his toys away to now, such as when he vacuums the house for an allowance, he is given the opportunity to learn how a business is managed and how to work for someone else to obtain an income. It is my dream for him to own his own business instead of working for others, but that's just my dream.

Either way, I am teaching him the value of becoming financially competent, responsible and, most of all, give him the freedom to dream about his future education and career. I often give him five one-dollar bills and let him divide it three ways using the envelope system taught by Dave Ramsey™. For the giving envelope, he learns to give his tithe back to God. I believe it all comes from God anyway. The saving envelope is for money to invest at the bank, and the spending envelope is to purchase any toy of his choice, based on my approval. In doing this, I know I have hope that when I die, I can leave my hard-earned dollars in capable hands.

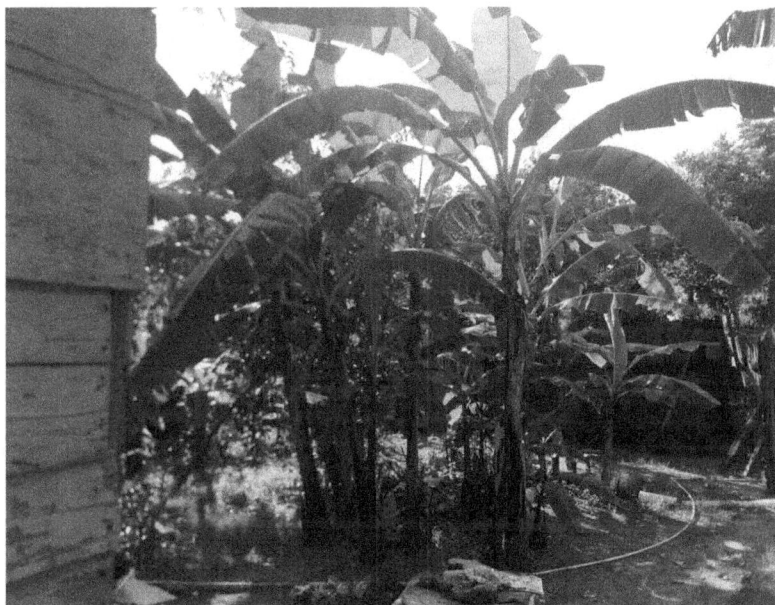

Image 3: *Banana tree. Our main source of green bananas.*

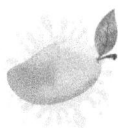

Power Thought

A family that works together can stay together and be successful. From a young age, I learned that unity is powerful. I would not have been able to have a second income if my sister Gina was not able to help me build my house in Jamaica. I have peace inside knowing that if I were to die today, my little Nathan, hopefully, will be financially fine. I believe that leaving something for your kids to stand on is so refreshing. I've taught him how to handle money in ways that will flow into adulthood. I pray he will not squander what I leave him. He can build on it and make his mama proud. My heart smiles as I imagine this.

If I could change one thing about my father's way of thinking, it would be his views about investment. With abundant thinking it is often said that it's not what you earn but what you save. If my father had budgeted his money to cover his expenses until his next salary was paid, then he could have had a little more to spend. There would be no interest payments. If he had also refrained from consuming so much alcohol with friends, he could have saved all that money and preserved his health. I don't want my culture to cancel those types of *ifs* in their lives; I want them to wake up, prevent it, think, and do it right.

But life's lessons, as we all know, come in various forms. This was the lesson I had to learn to escape this misguided cultural mindset. My father did not live from paycheck to paycheck. He lived worse. I interpret living paycheck to paycheck as the money I earn this week helping me to survive until the next paycheck is ready. But no, my father went and credited food supplies, thus taking away from his income before he received it in his hands. He was living beyond his means, above his income, so nothing was left for investments, security, or emergencies for his large family.

I hurt sometimes when I remember Shelly getting an asthma attack. She would sit in the tripod position—a position where the back is arched to allow for maximum lung expansion. I watched her as she struggled to breathe, her eyes popping wide with fear and panic. The inability of my parents to afford to take her to the hospital because we had no money is upsetting. Instead, various herbs were boiled and given to her in hopes she would get better.

These herbs damaged my sister's teeth. There was a myth they applied in one of their "cures," where Shelly walked around a banana tree while my father chopped the top off the tree. The belief was that this would get rid of the asthma. It did not. That was dangerous, too, as the machete could have accidentally cut my sister. Thinking about this fills me full of rage and makes me more determined than ever to be able to be financially stable enough to have access to competent medical care.

I learned from watching the way that borrowed money impacted us. The practice creates a feeling of hopelessness and feeds into the insecurity that there will never be enough because you don't, or never will, have the means to pay it back. Now, I refuse to pay interest; I refuse to participate in paying back loans that I can do without. Looking back at these life lessons teaches me to avoid borrowing money, to live on a budget and spend far less than I earn, and at the end of it, there is a brighter light than the Jamaican pension plan I grew up with. I like the idea where my money will take care of me (not Nathan's money but the fruit of my investments that multiply) while I sleep peacefully.

Chapter 6

Poverty Mindset

My mother's level of education ended at the elementary stage. Can you imagine the low income that "took care of" our large family? My father did all types of odd jobs to feed us and his girlfriends. Remember, he had twenty-three of us of who I am aware of. My mother was not the only mother. Before my mother met my father, he had eight kids with one woman and then four more kids with four other women. Two of my sisters from these twelve died. All the others are still living today. My mother had eleven of the twenty-three children. Two died in childbirth and Paul and Wayne died in their twenties and thirties because they choose to take up guns and steal. They wanted to satisfy their lack of resources by taking away people's hard-earned money without working honestly for it. It does not pay to be a "bad man." This will obviously end your life.

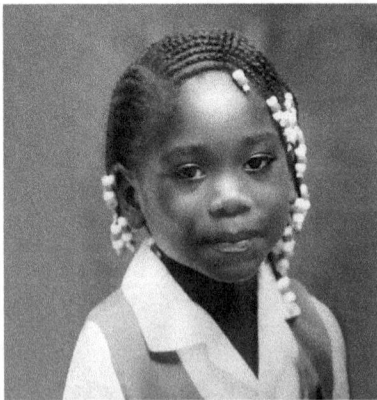

Image 4: Marie recalls her story. This child climbed the almond tree to see what was going on with her brother.

During one discussion, my sister Marie shared the story with me of a time when members in the community came looking for our brother Taddy, armed with sticks and stones. To me, he was not a bad man; he was just Taddy, my brother.

"Marie, tell me what happened that day," I said.

"I was alerted when I heard one of my sisters say, 'Mama, dem come fi Taddy.' [Mama, they are coming for Taddy]. Yes, that day the community people came looking for Taddy because he stole something. I can't recall what, but I can remember climbing the big almond tree in the side of our yard. Remember that tree, Sherene (my nickname)?"

"Yeah, I remember. We would sometimes sleep up there because that passion fruit tree would grow and intertwine with the branches of the almond tree, creating a bed to lie on. We were skin and bones then, so we were safe." We both chuckled.

"But Marie, weren't you scared?"

"I was terrified, but with the homes being separated by the zinc fence, the only way to see what was going on in Jim Brown's yard was to go high up the tree." Marie contorted her face and said with emphasis as she remembered, "These people were trying to kill my brother!" In a calmer tone, she continued. "And at the same time, I did not want to get in trouble, but I had to see."

"What do you mean, you did not want to get in trouble? And why were they looking for him in Jim Brown's yard?"

"Because he lived there for a while. Papa could not take it anymore with Taddy, so he had to leave."

"I did not know that he lived there. All I can remember is being hungry."

"Papa was trying to protect us from the stress that comes with Taddy."

"Yeah, Papa and his girls. I loved that man. Now tell me why you were in fear."

"I was fearful because I did not want the people to see me and then come to hurt me. And at the same time, I wanted to make sure that my brother was kept safe. I did not want to lose him. A lot of different emotions were going through my mind."

"How old were you, Marie?"

"About ten, I am not sure. This memory I cannot forget. It stayed with me because I was traumatized. Remembering him was always associated with some kind of fear. Never a really happy moment to recall, no laughter, just fear for him."

"Do you remember climbing the tree? I know it's a tree that we always climbed, but that day, was there anything in particular that changed in your style of climbing, I mean, did you go slower than usual?"

"I just remember I could not see what was happening. I was too small, and I could not get past the other family members. It was then that I got the idea to climb the tree, hoping to see what was happening."

"Marie, describe the mob."

"They had machetes, sticks, rocks, knives, and ice pricks [pick]." I remember the age of the ice prick, a well-known weapon causing many traumas, as was reported on the news. "Am telling you, but the people looked rugged; they were walking like they were mad. They were in their yard clothing, looking very disheveled, like they were working before they got the grand idea to chase down Taddy. They were angry and shouting 'Weh di bwoy deh?' [Where is the boy?]. No kids were in the mob, they were all young and old adults, male and female. Then I saw a glisten and I followed it, and there was Taddy with a silver gun in his hand in Mr. Bart's yard—the house beside Jim Brown's. Our eyes locked [mine and Taddy's] and he gestured with his finger to his lips to be quiet. But it was weird; nobody looked up, even though Jim Brown's house had no trees."

"Oh my."

"What amazed me more was the fact that the dogs in Mr. Bart's yard were not barking at Taddy. They were just lying there under the tree."

I remember Mr. Bart would feed us from the stale cake he collected (from the supermarkets in Spanish Town) that was to be thrown away. He would always come with his garbage truck and tell us to go search for the good cakes that had no fungus on them. Sometimes he would carry a few in his hands for us.

"Maybe the dogs knew him," I said.

The dogs in Jamaica are different from the dogs in America. They are only pets with their master. As a stranger, they will bite you—tear you to pieces—and the fault would be on you. That's the reason why I fear dogs up to today. I got attacked by a few and was bitten. It was not a good experience. All I was doing was walking in the lane, holding my fish. I think that day I ran faster than Usain Bolt to get rid of them.

"Maybe, but I was scared for my brother. They looked in Jim Brown's house—no Taddy; the goat pen—no Taddy; then they made their way to The Commons. I started to relax. They did not dare come to our house."

We had dogs, and Papa would not tolerate such nonsense. Taddy brought Mama a lot of stress. Not just Mama, *all of us*. But I miss his smile. He had evenly white teeth, hair that was always neatly combed with his pick comb, which he kept in his back pocket, and a kerchief in the other. His clothing was always neatly pressed. He was immaculate.

"But later that day," said Marie, "I recall the police coming and saying he stole from a woman. They barged into the house with their guns, turning over the mattress, pushing things out of the way. I felt ashamed because of how shabby the bed looked uncovered. Then Mama was walking behind them crying, saying '*My son did nothing*. He was with us all night.' I don't know if Taddy was with us or not, but that was what she said."

"I don't recall that part."

"I guess it was just where we were at the time. But Mama got so fed up with this that one day she held her arms up in the air and with tears in her eyes she cried out, 'God, I cannot take this anymore. Get him out of my sight!' I know there is a God because after that plea, about a week later, I never saw Taddy again. Mama's cup was running over with grief. I remember how contorted her face was and the tears running down her face as she bent over in despair. A mother who loves her children, her personal old age pension, asked God to remove her son from her presence."

Since then, we have not seen him, but someone from time to time would come by the house and say they spotted Taddy somewhere. All I know is, God answers prayer. Taddy was just gone. He disappeared without a trace.

Another discussion with my other sister Gina recalls part of the same incident.

"Gina, tell me your account of the time the community came after Taddy with sticks and stones."

"I remember soldiers and police coming from both entrances to the house—the lane and from The Commons—all coming in search of Taddy. It was a Sabbath morning. All the neighbors came out and were looking. It was a big scene. It was a sad morning."

"Why?"

"We were not used to this. They had big, long guns and pointed them at us. They came barging into the yard and pointed the guns."

"Did they really point the guns at us?" I asked disbelievingly.

"Yes, they did. Taddy was a notorious bad man, and they were scared. After a while, they lowered the guns because all they saw were a lot of children. Dem [they] pointed up dem [their] guns, but because of a bad man, they had their guns on cock because Taddy was the bad man. His name was up in di [the] station all di [the] time. They searched the house, throwing things here and there. Then they claimed they found a gun in the cane field."

"Did you see it?" I asked in shock.

"Yes, it was a small, black gun. I am not sure if they planted it, but that's what they said. Taddy had to go; we could not manage him. That morning Mama had to get a lawyer. Every time Taddy got in trouble, she was always getting him out. They always win. I don't know where she got money for a lawyer, but Taddy was always getting off. She can explain herself and, in her eyes, Taddy was never wrong. But he was so finger fearing (take what is not yours)," Gina said in frustration. "He was very slick. He would not get caught. It was just too much. I have to go watch the news. Later."

Gina does not like to recall the sad days. As an older child, she recalls more, and she experienced the hunger more. She is usually very strong, but when it comes to those memories, she tries to avoid them. A few days later, she remembered other details.

"I can't blame Taddy for interfering with other people because he would take people's things and then come and cook for us. He would catch the fish from the pond in the front of the yard, but he would give according to how you behave. Marie would not get any because she would talk and tell Papa how Taddy caught the fish out of the pond. Shelly would always get some because she was always sick with her asthma, so she didn't talk much. You would get some because you didn't talk either, or the same with Suzan. Taddy saved us a lot."

"How did that pond come about?"

"Taddy would catch the fish from the wastewater pond over at Ebony and come to cook. Papa saw them and decided he would dig a pit like the one for the pit toilet. In it he put the baby ones and let me tell you sumting [something] Sherene, dat [that] fishpond gave us a lot of fish over the years."

"Hmm, hmmm," I said in agreement.

"You were so tough. You at school, you stay hungry, yuh nuh [you never] cry. And as you come home, yuh [you] find ockro and the yam head and you cooked. Even the ackee you fried up with butter. I don't know how you did it, but sumting yuh [something you] always found to cook. We always had you or Taddy to save our lives. From you going to Miss Lue, you were different. Taddy's not here, maybe I cannot honor him, but I wish I can honor you one day."

I thought about what Gina said about Taddy and me. I recall a few moments with Taddy, but I was never really in tune with him. I recall that I was just too hungry to focus on anything else. It could have been the age difference. Taddy would not give Marie food when he cooked because she was a tattletale, yet she protected him from the mob. The power of kinship stands taller than our moments of anger and disagreement. It leads us to do what is not ethical at times to protect those we love. Is it wrong? Is it right? But why does it have to be a situation where it's right or wrong? Can't we say that because it is survival for basic needs that hunger is the exception? Some people might agree. But wrong is wrong, that's the thing.

A Walk in My Shoes
by Delpha Clarke

Had you walked in my shoes,
you'd notice there is no outer or inner sole.
I used my socks for soles,
the upper straps on top to make them whole.
Had you shaken my hands, you'd feel how coarse they were
from the hard work
of rearing, cleaning, and plucking chickens.
Had you walked in my shoes,
you'd notice we used to be the same.
Try walking in my shoes
before you decide to end my trodding,
to kill me for what little I have.
Don't you see? I used to think like you.
If you'd walk in my new shoes,
you'd see that you can exceed beyond where I am now.

I dedicate this poem to my brother Taddy and those who choose crime to feed their hunger. The fear I have about landing in poverty, now that I've left, is the same fear that continues in my culture. Nothing was handed down to me from parents, government, or anyone else. Has anything been handed down to you? Jamaicans, I challenge you to put the guns down and take up a book instead. I dare you to dream and take action. Learn how to change your mindset. Let my story inspire you to make a choice to change your thinking and choose a better life.

My mother was not able to look after us when she was at work, so the bigger set of kids would take care of the younger ones. The end result of this was that some of us were not educated or able to pursue the career of our dreams. The cycle of poverty continued. Heck, I wanted to become an astronaut. I knew I would become one if I could just figure out how to get out of Jamaica, get some money, or even find someone to talk to and show me how, but I was too busy trying to figure out whether we were going to have dinner that night or not.

In survival mode, we thought about simple things such as, *How do I get through today?* or, *Where will dinner be coming from tonight?* I had no extra time to dream of endless possibilities. *No, not today. Today, I can only feel the worms grumbling in my belly.* But I let them grumble because I had nothing to feed them except water, which we had in abundance. But drinking water made my empty stomach hurt more. Have you ever tried drinking water on a hungry belly? I'm not talking about two or three hours of hunger. I am talking about days of hunger before a piece of food gets to your mouth, which was not even a belly full. The water just filled a temporary gap. When the water hit the top of my stomach, the cramps that followed felt deadly, sometimes crippling, to the point where I had to bend over and hug my stomach. The worms in my belly got louder. Not to mention the unbearable headaches.

When this subsided, I would get desperate and walk barefoot, digging my toes in the loose dirt in my backyard, praying to find buried money. One day I recall finding two dollars. I leaped for joy and ran to Miss Fatty to purchase a bulla cake; vanilla, nutmeg, sugar, and sometimes ginger all mixed with flour. I salivated as I took a huge bite and let it linger to savor every spice. They don't make bulla cake as good now as they did back then. I was in bulla heaven. Hunger made me selfish. I did not want to share my bulla cake with my tribe, so I hid it to consume all by myself in private. If I shared, there would not be enough, and I would still be hungry. The worms would only settle temporarily. I wanted to feel full and stay full, if only for one day or as long as it lasted. Then, I felt guilty after my belly was full, but I swore God buried those two dollars for me that day. The truth is, I knew He would want me to share. My father always taught us that food was for sharing; we eat and then we pass it out the other end. The latter was never said very politely.

All of us grew up with that mentality of sharing our food supplies. I don't know how to sit and wait for a man to provide for me. I didn't have a government that gave me welfare or was willing to send me to school. All I had was a sense of survival, a brain that I used the best way I knew how—to eat and to get to where I am today.

This way of life left me asking myself the questions: When will I stop working so hard and learn to relax and breathe at this stage in my life? or, If I stop working this hard, will I go back to my old state of poverty? and When will I learn to accept a gift without feeling awkward because I did not sweat for it?

I never want to experience that side of poverty in my life again. But you would think that a sensible person such as myself should not give so much until I have built a foundation that I can stand on—one that won't crumble later. When I think about what I went through because we had no money, I ask myself why I would not give to others to either stop or prevent someone else from going through what I went through. Man, it just hurts too much when I remember what hunger felt like. I know I can give more later on if I am able to stand up and extend a hand without falling down.

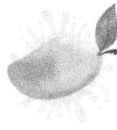

Power Thought

Out of the twenty-three of us, only two became bad men. We all had similar teachings using the same classroom, yet two strayed from the tribe. Taddy lived with us, but Wayne lived with his father in the inner city of Kingston. The two were close. Wayne got shot while trying to rob someone of his chain on a bus. A harmed police officer in Mufti was traveling, unbeknownst to Wayne. Nothing came of the incident. Another thief went six feet under while the mother mourned and struggled to find money to bury her son.

We can say poverty led to their demise or can ask why they could not have been satisfied with the little we had, just like the rest of us. Why could we not work together and unite our resources, be it in physical strength or whatever special talent each of us had, to get out of poverty? Why did my father not think to purchase land to leave for his kids in-stead of having a dozen women? And the whys continue in my head. I could say the answer to some of these questions is that it was due to him being uneducated, but education comes in several forms.

I have this burning desire today to have a business owned and operated by the Clarke family. Unity is strength. America is great because all the states have combined their resources. We can all be great if we all work together as one. In the emergency room, we say that teamwork makes the dream work. Life is much easier with this mindset.

After the abolition of slavery, the Black man did not yet know how to be free. He did not receive the same level of education as those who formerly oppressed him. Even though he was physically free, he was still as oppressed mentally as those who feared the threat of even considering their equality. My opinion is that the oppression equaled a poverty mindset because the lack of education left the Black man to fend for himself. Without education, it took longer for him to find his value as a human being.

Some of us had sense enough to start reading and learning how to do more than survive. Some of us watched how others lived, while people like myself had a burning desire to dare to want more than what I was born into.

That desire drove me out of my misguided cultural mindset, on to an education and upward to a better life. I have a plan, and I have stayed committed to that plan.

Chapter 7

Mama Recalls

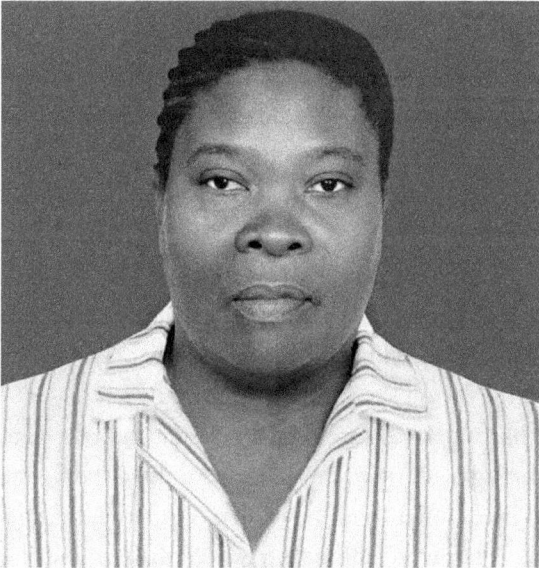

Image 5: *Mama.*

I asked my mother to tell me her story, and these are her words. "I was baptized at the Spanish Town Seventh Day Adventist church. When my youngest daughter, Marie, was three months old. Miss Kathrine took me to the Spanish Town Hospital when I had my nervous breakdown. I was taking my clothes off on the road in public. I was [mentally] sick. I could not take care of Marie. I had to send for my niece Dion to take care of Marie."

"Why did you get a nervous breakdown, Mama?" I asked.

"I believe that hard work and having so many children contributed to my nervous breakdown. Despite my being sick, I still had to work. When I got sick Marie was three months old. I was not even able to sit up on my bottom. God, I just thank you; I just thank you because if it were not for you, I would not be here today.

Marie's head came down in the right position, but this baby would not deliver. The nurse left me three times and still no baby. She had to hold me in the soft part of my stomach and press down to push Marie out."

"What did you have to tell yourself?"

"It was all pain. It is like I was sitting on Marie. I had to tell myself that I had to live. Thank you, Jesus. I am telling you, Sherene, God was working in my life even though I did not know."

I asked my mother at some point why she did not use contraceptives after having problems during pregnancy. She said she used them once for three months and threw them out because she did not want anything to damage her body. After having Marie, she prayed and told God she wanted no more because she had almost died. Marie was her last child. God answered her prayer. My mother saw God as a means of escape from the prison she was in with my father.

"Dion had to bathe Marie, comb her hair, and take care of her every day. Dion brought Marie to my bedside for me to hold. She was pretty, had a lot of hair on her head. Dion always put a red ribbon in her hair. Dion washed all of your clothes and carried them to Judith to be ironed and returned with them for school the next Monday morning.

"When I took sick and could not help myself, Judith and my mother came [for a visit] one Sunday morning. When my mother saw me she said, 'It is not you going to bury me, but I will bury you.' Judith told me that she was a member of the First Day Adventist church in Kingston. Judith and my mother prayed for me that Sunday morning. They took me outside and circled a sheet around me. They gave me a bush bath that Sunday morning.

"I decided that morning I was going to go to your sister's church and give my life to Jesus and get baptized. The Monday morning afterward, Sister Dennis Langley came by. She was a nurse who always took care of me at the clinic. When she saw that I was sick—'Whoa!' the sister exclaimed. And she sat down and talked to me. I said to her, 'Nurse

Langley, I am going to get baptized at my daughter's church. One Brother McBean from the Seventh Day Adventist church in Spanish Town
came to visit me twice before I got sick. He told me about the Seventh
Day Adventist message.' I said to her, 'I love the Adventist message, and
I am going to my daughter's church.' She said, 'I like how you like the
Adventist message—don't change it [your mind]—the Adventist church
is God's true church on earth. She asked me if I wanted her to send a
Bible worker to study the Word with me. She sent the Bible worker to
me one day in the week. [One day], I saw a lady and when she came by,
she said, 'Good morning, Sister Langley sent me.' She said her name was
Sister Jackson from the Seventh Day Adventist church. Sister Jackson
studied and visited with me.

"When Marie was four months old, I started to visit the Spanish
Town Seventh Day Adventist church. I took Dingy—your brother, and
Donna, your sister. I got baptized at this church and so did Dingy.

"When I left Jobe's Lane and moved to Redpond, I met Sister Joyce
Rotham from the Saint John's Seventh Day Adventist church. That lady
and her husband taught me a lot. She took me all around. She took
me up in the hills of Saint Catherine to do missionary work, all over in
Spanish Town. Wow, we had good times together."

"Why did you move from Job's Land to Redpond?"

"Ivan said that he did not want to live on any free land because he
wanted to plant his ground provision."

"Mama, tell me how it went with the children."

"When I started to attend Saint John's SDA, I took all of you with
me to church and baptized all of you, one and two together. Everyone
became a member of the Saint John's SDA church. Thank God, praise
you Jesus. So, everyone stayed in the church except for Donna and Dingy."

"Really, Mama, Donna was baptized?"

"Yes, Donna baptized with all of you until everybody grew up and
the rest of you were still in the church."

"How did going to church affect your life?"

"After I accepted Christ as my personal Savior, it was wonderful. Even now, I know God holds the future. The Seventh Day Adventist church is God's church, and I will always worship and fellowship here until God calls me home. I am in America now and I still love to worship at an SDA church. It is God's true church. To know God for yourself is a wonderful thing, and I will continue to lift up the name of Jesus until I die.

"Every one of my children was baptized into the SDA church except Taddy, who was a bad boy, running up and down all over the place. It is so sweet to trust in Jesus. Just to take him at his Word, just to rest upon his promises, just to know this says the Lord. To be with Christ is a wonderful life to live. Being with Jesus Christ is wonderful, praise God.

"Oh, Sherene, before I got baptized, I remember one night in my sleep I dreamed I saw water—a wide river, and when I looked into the water, it was pretty—even the stones were beautiful. When I looked straight before me, I saw a lady in full white, from head to toe. And she said to me, 'Would you like to come across?' I said yes. As she put her foot in the water, I awoke out of my sleep."

"Mama, what do you think this dream meant?"

"I believe that dream was a good dream for me at that time. I believe that dream represented my baptism."

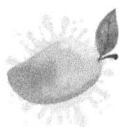

Power Thought

Your legacy can be whatever you want it to be. Your family is a part of you, but your belief systems and habits can change as you grow up, and grow older.

Even though I speak with so much passion about how I grew up, I have a lot of compassion toward my family because we had a good fam-

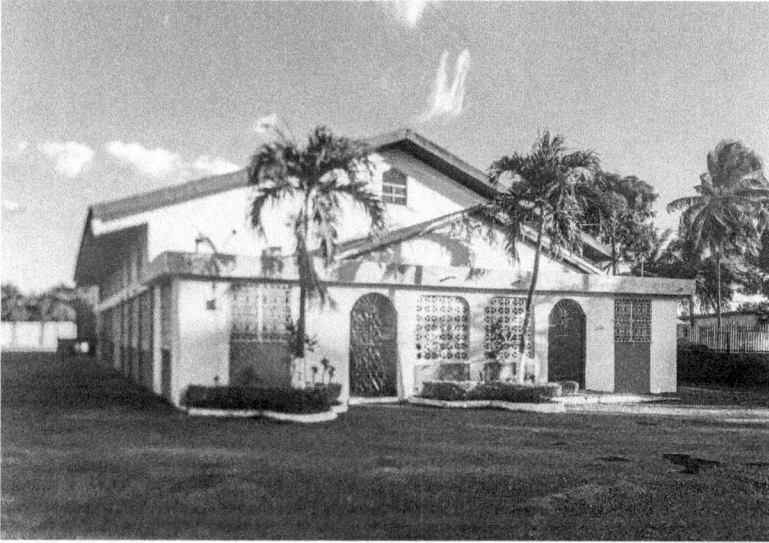

Image 6: Current picture of church.

ily bond. There was a lot of good that came out of it. Mama just did not know any different, but her love for us was unquestionable.

Your beliefs, your customs, and your dreams are part of who you are. They provide contentment and courage to face another day. If you did not have a stable childhood or you do not have positive memories, you can create your own.

Chapter 8

Let the Children Play

*D*espite the struggles, Jamaica was beautiful to me because as siblings, we had some fun times. Nathan is lonely because he is an only child. Looking back, I compare my vibrant, loud childhood to his, and there are times I feel as if he's missing out. I try to teach him some of the simple games we played as children. We played music, usually Kenny Rogers or Bob Marley, and danced every Sunday morning when it was cleaning-up time. We could not dance the dancehall style, but we did our thing. We would play dolly house and cooked callaloo soup—cut from the wild bush growing in the yard. We made kites from book leaves and sticks—from the trees around us. We knew how to make mats from old clothing. It was fun to sit at night and do this while talking and laughing. We played Piece is Mine when we ate. One could join the game by overlapping the pinky finger with each other. Whenever dinner was served and two of our fingers were not overlapping and we called you out, that meant a piece of what you were eating was now mine. This was fun for us. We climbed trees and played water wars. The best part of it was in the evenings, when we would all go out in the same open field and pick up cow dung, which we used to make mosquito fires. Nathan thinks this is 'yucky,' but it was fun for us. During the summer, our brothers came over to teach us marble games. In December, we had sodas. This was the only time we got this to drink. We would keep the empty bottles all day.

We did not receive gifts as children. We did not know to miss gifts, nor what it was like to receive them, and we loved that we had each other. This is the greatest gift that one can possess—having a family. There is nothing like the feeling of having an entire tribe that has your back. That's the feeling of my family. I would give them up for nothing or no one in this world. We grew up with so much love to give, and we only asked that it was not abused.

Stucky (Jamaican Tag)

I could see the wind blowing through the grass as I mapped out the direction for how I could speed my way out. Donna, Marie, and Gena were spread across the vital areas where I could make my escape and return to the ring. Shelly and Susan gathered around me closer in the ring, whispering.

"Sherene, you may need to go through the grass."

"No, I cannot. We will lose points if we go out of bounds there. All I can do is the zigzag motion."

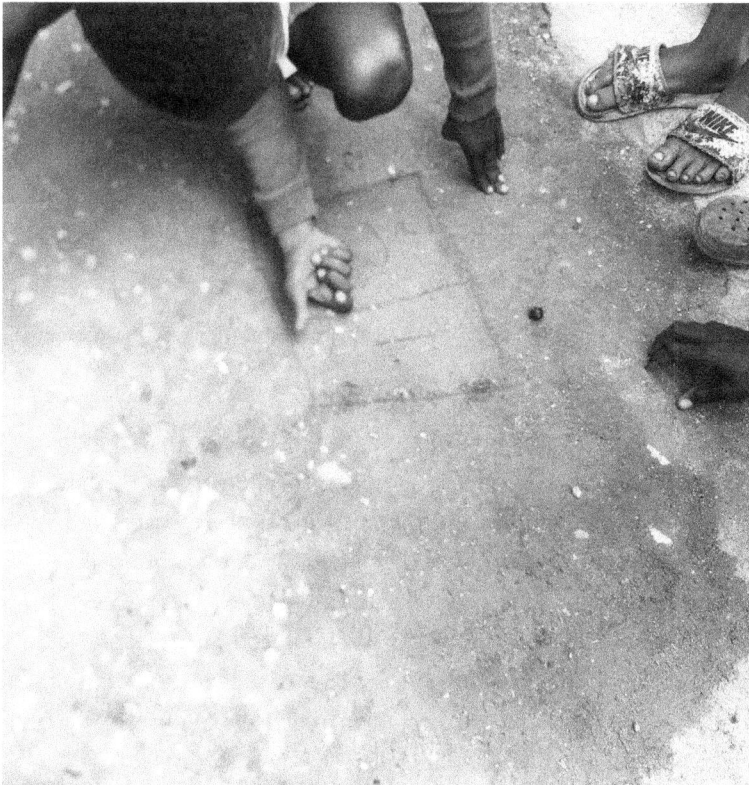

Image 7: Kids gather in the lane to play marble.

I ran out of the ring, trying to evade my opponent. I zigzagged across The Commons, jumped over a rock, and breathlessly looked over my shoulder to see Marie lagging. I laughed because I was not going to be caught, only to feel a slap on my hand and Gena saying, "Got you."

Now I was stuck. I knew I could not move unless one of my partners in the ring came and unfroze me, hence the name "Stucky." Sometimes when I was "unstuck," we'd both try to return to the ring or else be caught by our opponents. This was a game that required speed with stealth. I loved it because I was usually the fastest one in the group, but Gena had stealth. I liked it when we were on the same team because we usually won with our combined skills. This was one of our favorite games.

Sightings

This game was usually played in The Commons and required three to four players. Sometimes it would be me, Suzan, Marie, and Gena. Shelly was too sick (asthma), and the others would claim that they were too old or busy. When it was four of us, we partnered up, Marie at one end and Gena at the other. I stood in the middle and tried to dodge the ball being thrown by either Marie or Gena. The object of the game was to not allow the ball to touch you. When that happened, you were out of the game. Then it was your partner's turn. When all of the members on one team were out, the other team got their turn.

Elastic

This game requires less physical activity and could be played indoors. All we needed was a wall to bounce the elastic bands from. The farther the bounce, the harder it was to overlap with another elastic band. When there was an overlap, you'd win that set. This game was often played with my brothers as it was not considered a girl game.

In the same open field, we played hopscotch, marble, cricket, baseball, Ludo, and many more games, some of which, I attempt to teach Nathan. We had no tablets or phones to damage our eyes. We grew up on the land, figuratively and literally.

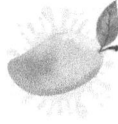

Power Thought

Let us start showing appreciation for family and friends. When we are down, they are there. Let's cherish them in the happy times as well and build each other up. Sometimes just let your hair down and listen to music and dance your crazy dance, forgetting your troubles, even if it is for a minute. This is refreshing to the soul. In your life, and in mine, it feels impossible not to remember the continuous loop of childhood insults, stings, or hurts can feel impossible, but we must. We must set it aside and forget those things we've allowed to remain in us, and instead create our new story and identity. It is the only way forward.

Let us teach our children more outdoor games. Get them accustomed to physical activity so that when they grow into adulthood, they will be healthier and able to fight off lifestyle diseases such as high blood pressure and diabetes. Let the games begin.

Chapter 9

Education

I was one of the fortunate of the brothers and sisters who went straight from primary (what we call elementary school in America) through to university. I say fortunate because not all my brothers and sisters were able to do so. The eldest sibling had to stay at home to take care of the younger ones. The Jamaican government system makes it compulsory for children to attend school, but these laws were not strictly practiced—this was the norm in some households. In the church, we have the Ten Commandments that provide guidance and basically point out our sins. To obey them is a choice given by God. We had the laws of the land that told us we must send our kids to school. Based on my experience, children must be fed before going to school in the morning to give them the best advantage for learning. In our case, we often did not have food in the morning.

Despite my brothers and sisters not getting a formal education, they were all street-smart and used that to survive. They have done more than survive. Each one of them owns their own home today. Some have more than the others and manage rental properties. In Jamaica, this is known as prosperity. People who know us talk about our progressive mentality. A builder once looked at me while he was building Gina's house and said, "Your time is coming soon."

I laughed.
"You don't believe me. Watch and see," he said.

He was right. Our family principle was where each one of us would come behind and help the others build their own homes. The man recognized that my day to have my own home would come soon. Our family does not believe in renting. My mother's principle lives on in me— we were nurtured by her to not borrow, beg, or go to people's houses for food or shelter. She emphasized that we be proud of the little we might have and to work with it. I disagreed with my husband when he bought a kiddie Timex watch for my Nathan's seventh birthday; it is the type that can be used to track Nathan, text, or call others. He said he bought it for him because he does not want him to feel inferior or left out when he is around his peers. Really. He passed his fears and insecurities on to Nathan. I want Nathan to be an independent, strong-minded, intelligent young man who thinks for himself and is not influenced by others. I keep telling him to be a leader and not a follower. I need him to not want things just because others have them. I want him to learn to be creative and content with who he is and what he has. I want him to prepare for the windows and doors that open for him so he may pursue his dreams with confidence, and with assurance that he can do what he wants to do in this life. The sky is not the limit for him because there is no limit, and this is what I want him to know. According to my broth-er-in-law, it's just the view, meaning that his possibilities far exceed his view of the sky, illustrating the endless possibilities that one can achieve if they are willing to push forward in achieving their goals.

My eldest sister, Judith, from my mother's side of the family, had a CVA. While I was working in the emergency room one day, a nurse came up to me and said, "Delpha, we have your sister in Room 59, and we had to call a stroke alert on her." The news paralyzed me for a minute. I thought the worst as I walked to her room, as we so often do at times. I wondered if she might be paralyzed, die, or be able to speak normally—oh, my heart was in pain. My eyes teared up when I saw her lying in the bed with her face twisted to one side as she spoke. I started to cry. I rushed toward her and gave her a hug. She started to cry, as did her husband. My thoughts battered me as I continued to wonder why

I didn't tell her to slow down or stop working so hard. I should have invited her out to have some fun.

Why do we immediately start talking down to ourselves, questioning our actions when tragedy strikes?

I dried my tears and walked to the CT [scan] room with her. As we transferred her to the table, I teared up again. I had to walk out and find a corner to shed my tears.

I keep telling Nathan, "Don't cry first, try and solve your problems and then cry." By the time he is finished solving the problem, there will be no reason for tears. Yet here I was crying my eyes out and I could not solve the problem at first. I wanted my sister Judith here, healthy and strong, for we still had a lot to accomplish. As one of the older siblings who did not go to school, she took care of us when I was younger. She looked out for me. She still looks out for me now, as I write these words. She gave me my first new suit. On her first trip to Panama, she bought clothing to sell. She was known as a higgler. That's the local term in Jamaica for someone who buys and sells clothing. My new suit was black and white with a gold band around the neckline. I dressed up that Sabbath morning for church feeling very happy and sharp; I was ready to take on the world. This time I was going to church not dressed in someone else's clothing but my own. I was always thankful when I received clothing from other church members, but feeling sharp in my very own suit was invigorating.

People around could see me cry. Maybe they were wondering why I was crying when it was just a mild stroke. I did not see this. I just saw all the limitations that this could place on Judith. (She is 99 percent better now, thank God.) My coworkers comforted me, but they didn't know our history and they didn't understand my tears, which reminds me of the understanding of angels. The songwriter Johnson Oatman wrote a hymn in 1894 called "Holy, Holy Is What the Angels Sing," and in it, the angels can only stand and listen to the song of the redeemed. They cannot join the singing of the happy, blood-washed throng, which sounds like the sound of many waters, because they are not mortal.

We can sing about great trials, battles fought, and victories won, and praise our great Redeemer, who says "Well done." Another part we sing is about how the angels will fold their wings when we sing redemption's song, for angels have never felt the joys that our salvation brings. The angels cannot join the song because they have not lived in the saints' shoes.

Neither the nurses nor the angels understand the trials my sisters and I had growing up. They don't know about the nights we went to bed hungry or to school without breakfast, about not having proper clothing or even underwear to put on. We had no lotion to oil our skin and used the bar soap at times to create some kind of sheen on our legs. They don't know about the things we did not accomplish. Judith and I had plans to visit the very beautiful parts of Jamaica, the parts that tourists visit. We were going to live it up, so to speak, as we were not able to see these places when we were younger. This same sister taught me to share and not be selfish. You could see this in the way she treated others. She lived what she preached.

Growing up in a poverty-stricken community in Jamaica, the ghetto, as we called it, young girls became pregnant and withdrew from school. In this third world country, we had no schools for the pregnant teenagers who happened to fall into this trap. One classmate of mine got pregnant in third form (in America, this is the ninth grade), and she had to stop going to school. I saw her a few months later selling in the Town, trying to survive. Her education was terminated. To make the situation even worse was that some of these girls' "baby daddies" left them sometimes before or after the child was born. I observed this and made a vow that this would not happen to me.

I experienced a life-sobering event when my sister got pregnant at the age of seventeen.

"Get out. You going bring shame down on the family."

As I remember, I looked at Suzan and her eyes were red with unshed tears. My mother was hard as steel, but she feared her other girls would fall into the same trap, and this was not allowed. Suzan went to live with Judith. This event scared us other girls, and I made sure to never let it happen to me. I never want the wrath of Mama upon me. People gossiped that this was going to happen to the rest of us; sadly, some of those people were from the church. Not everyone who claims they are a Christian is Christlike. There will be good and there will be bad everywhere you go. People in general seem to want to see you always down on your face when you are poor. People like feeding the poor but believe that those same poor people should remain poor. It's as if they are saying, "How dare you strive and become capable of managing yourself." Poverty transforms the mind into mental slavery. But if you don't know any different, you can only know it is something to escape through education and experiences outside of the home.

That is how they act. I was able to avoid boys more easily as I was not the first choice for them. I was too black, too skinny, and too ugly for the boys who wanted brown-skinned girls. Oh, how it amazed me sometimes because these brown-skinned girls could not even read. The slavery mentality still existed. We did not appreciate what we had or who we were as individuals or as a people. Yet the boys treated us that way.

One day I boarded a bus from Spanish Town to downtown Kingston, where I wanted to sell my hair scrunchies. I found a window seat and waited for the bus to fill with passengers before it would move.

"Man, how you so ugly?" a guy shouted from the window outside at the gentleman sitting in front of me. The gentleman did not respond. Not pleased that he did not evoke a response from him, he then turned to me and said,

"Hey, are you related to him?"

Repeatedly, I encountered these types of comments growing up. I cannot describe the hurt and pain I felt from those comments. Tears often flowed, but I knew I had to get past this. Over time, the words became a reality in my mind in a continuous loop.

We have a well-known musical artist in Jamaica by the name of Bob Marley. He was a conscientious singer. The words in his music often told the story of Jamaicans in the time we were living in. His songs are timeless. In one of his songs, he spoke about mental slavery, telling us to

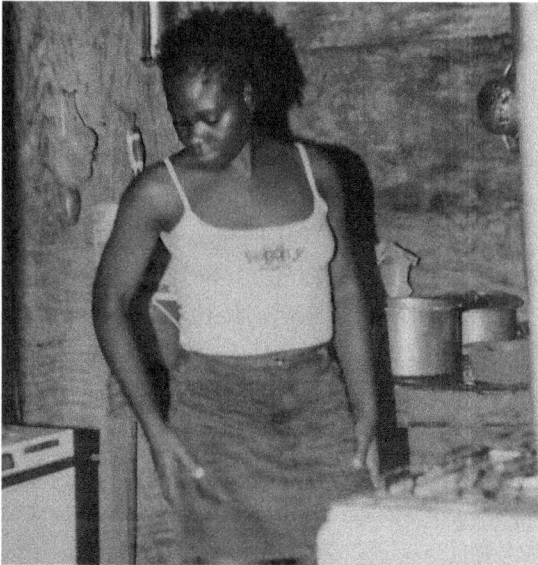

Image 8: Delpha in the kitchen contemplating what to cook for dinner.

emancipate ourselves from it because we are the only ones who can free our minds! This is a powerful statement.

On the slave plantation, strong, young, Black men were chosen and sent to sleep with other Black women so that the slave owner could increase his workforce. It did not matter if the women wanted it or not, for they had no voice. Today we are burdened to stand up for ourselves because we do have one. It is our responsibility, to create a better life!

We are no longer in slavery, but the mentality is still there. Some men now go around from woman-to-woman having children and walking out, not caring or fighting to maintain the relationship. This mentality included a preference for a lighter skin color—at one point in time, the perceived beauty preference was for lighter-skinned girls, who could be found working in the banks of Jamaica, where banking was considered a glamorous profession. These light-skinned girls often took their skin color for granted and did not study, assuming their looks would get them a job. This has changed. Now, when I visit a bank in Jamaica, I see almost the opposite. This is an improvement; the shackles that bind us are slowly being removed.

Bob Marley said none but us can free our minds. We need to condition ourselves as Black people to rise and emancipate ourselves from these thoughts. Anything that we condition the mind to, along with failure to break those chains, can be put in the class of mental slavery. Be it a slave to debts, a slave to sin, or a slave to being with an abuser., it's all up to us to get rid of the shackles. No one stands in our way but the person looking back at us in the mirror.

Once I learned that I had the freedom to choose my way out of my current status in life, I went to work to free myself from the oppression of poverty and replaced it with education and ambition. I just had to apply the new knowledge to my life. I grew up with this pervasive thought in my mind that I was not good enough for a man because I lacked these so-called looks. Yes, my thought process said that I did not have the looks, but how dare I not have the brains to become an intelligent woman. I developed this determination, this drive, this force to succeed at what I do.

One day, looks will fade away but my education will always be there. Looking at it from this perspective, I ask myself what I have to lose. Let's begin the fight. Even if I were ugly, I love me, so you better plan to love me too. These days, I am being me and I love who I am. Who am I to place a limit on myself?

At the age of twelve, I still did not know how to read. I was in a class where no one was able to. When you were behind, you were still placed on the same level as other children your age. You were not held back because you could not read, and they kept allowing us to move from one grade to the next despite this. Back in the '80s and '90s, students often graduated elementary school and high school without knowing how to read. (The system in Jamaica has now changed; you must be able to read to move forward.)

One day we got a new teacher. This teacher did not flog me. When I was in preschool, what we called basic school in Jamaica, I had a teacher who would walk with a red belt and flog me over the back every morning when trying to teach me to spell my name. I can vividly recall her face when she came in, in the mornings. There was determination and spitefulness there. This I did not understand; to this day I am puzzled. I can remember her wearing a black skirt and white blouse most mornings. She had natural hair, and she had a lot of pimples on her face. I cannot recall what my classroom looked like, or even the friends I had there. All the memories I had were of her. I would often tremble by just looking at her or knowing that she would be in class soon. She did not need to touch me for me to fear her. I was conditioned to be like this from the way she treated me. I hated preschool because of that red belt and how it stung across my back.

This new teacher was the opposite of my previous nightmare. I fell in love with her. She had a gift for teaching. She opened the windows of knowledge to me. I can recall praying several prayers to God so that he would teach me how to read. I believed that God sent her just for me. At the age of twelve, he decided that it was time for me to learn to read. This beautiful teacher loved when I talked about my religion. I told her what being a Seventh Day Adventist was like. I loved that she was so interested in my life. She would lean forward, form a fist, and place it under her chin to lean on, and just listen to me with a smile on her face. She was in no rush to go anywhere. At that moment I felt like the most important person in the world to her. One day, she wrote two very long words on the board.

"Class, what is this word?"

I looked at the first word and tried to sound it out. I broke up the word into groups of two letters at a time:

Ed no... E-DU-CA-TION. "EDUCATION!" I shouted.

"Yes, Delpha, education!" She smiled a broad smile. I could see how proud of me she was. "Okay, class, let's try the other word."

I can't recall what the other word was. I know I did not attempt to figure it out as I was very busy being in awe of myself. This teacher made me want to teach. To this day, I still want to teach. She was just so awesome. If only I could remember her name or see her again. I would hug her so tight.

I started reading the Bible in morning worship and leading out in song service. This is the lineup for my mother's daughters in descending order: Judith, Suzan, Gina, Shelly, Shereen (myself), and Marie. For family worship, this would be the order we were called in, in rapid sequence, except for the eldest. Like Judith, the other brothers and sisters were much older and lived on their own.

When I attended church, I would go up on the platform and read to the congregation. This helped me gain confidence with public speaking, but I was still scared and insecure. I had two male friends I often attended church with. They lived in the richer part of the community. I learned a lot from them. The church was the only place I socialized with others. The three of us were a pack. We went on church trips together, camping with the Pathfinder's group to learn about the stars in star study. In my teenage years, I went to visit the beautiful part of Jamaica, the parts that tourists are accustomed to. I remember going to Dunn's River Falls. My first time experiencing the Caribbean blue waters was just incredible. I could stand in the water and see my feet and the baby fishes swimming around them. I had so much fun that day. A lot of my family members were there. My mother sat on the sand and played. This was the first time I saw her really enjoying herself. It was an unforgettable day.

I was looking for a career. I had now graduated from high school and was still not sure of what I wanted to do. As a matter of a fact, I thought I would just continue the path, like my other sisters, of selling scrunchies downtown. This did not feel right. I wanted more. I did not like the fact that my upstanding friends would pass and see me selling on the street. I felt ashamed, but I had to do what I had to do. I could also see that they did not like what I was doing.

My father was very ill, and because of this, I decided that I would go into nursing. The healthcare system in my country is not as advanced or glamorous as those in a first world country. The nurses were overworked and greatly underpaid. At that time, I could only think of one thing and that was to help him, so I started nursing school at the age of twenty-one. My father believed that education stopped at high school. I knew that by getting an education, this was the only way I would get out of my life of destitution. Also, I was going to help my father by joining the system to become a registered nurse.

Prior to leaving home, my sister informed me that she was scared about me going off to college as she was not sure how she was going to eat. At the time I had a small chicken farm that I would sell chicken from to bring additional income for rent. Every available family member helped. All the brothers, cousins, and sisters came together. Papa made a huge wood fire in the yard with three huge rocks to hold a zinc or oil drum that he had cut in half. A table was set up to chop the neck of each chicken off. When they stopped flopping their wings, we dipped them in the boiling water just long enough to pluck the feathers without damaging the skin. The finishing touch was done by Mama as she took off the fine hairs. With no hair remaining, I would gut the chicken, removing everything from the inside. The gizzard and liver were sold, as well as the feet of the chicken.

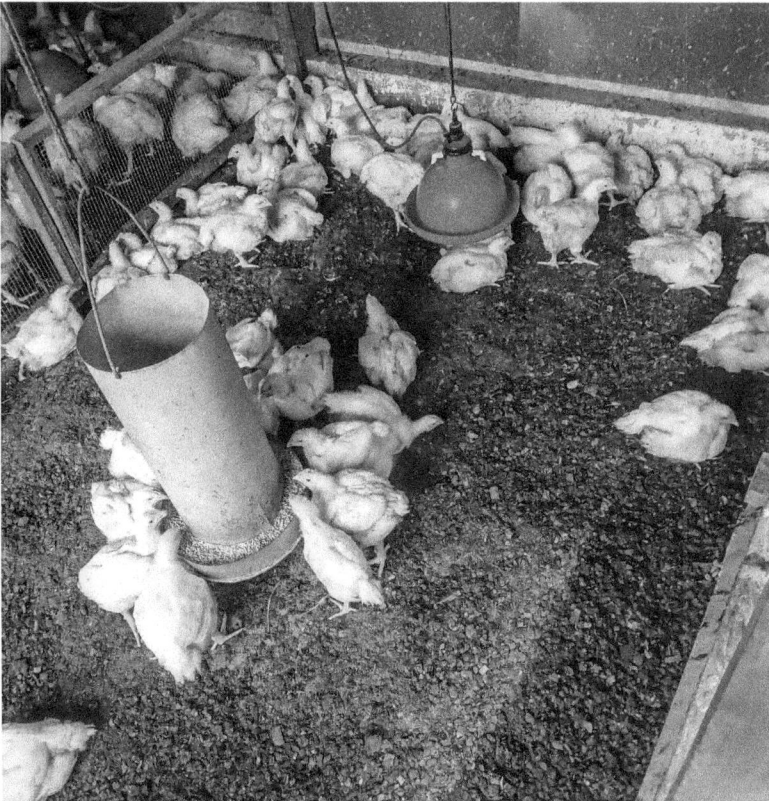

Image 9: Chickens feeding. They served as a form of income to assist in attending university. (2001).

I wanted to help Gina avoid hunger. On my last day, I filled the fridge with meat to hopefully last her until I got back home on break from university. I wished for this, but the university was miles away and the meat could not have lasted her that long. The savings that I carried over from my chicken rearing business got me started on paying my own rent and buying my own food.

Those four years of nursing school were challenging. I remember getting out of bed to join the long lines at the student loan bureau. Every year I applied for a loan, except for the final year (Suzan paid my tuition that year). I got through without hesitation. The loan bureau would only qualify those who were destitute, and I mean destitute by the fact that I used outdoor toilets and lived in a boarded house with a zinc roof. We

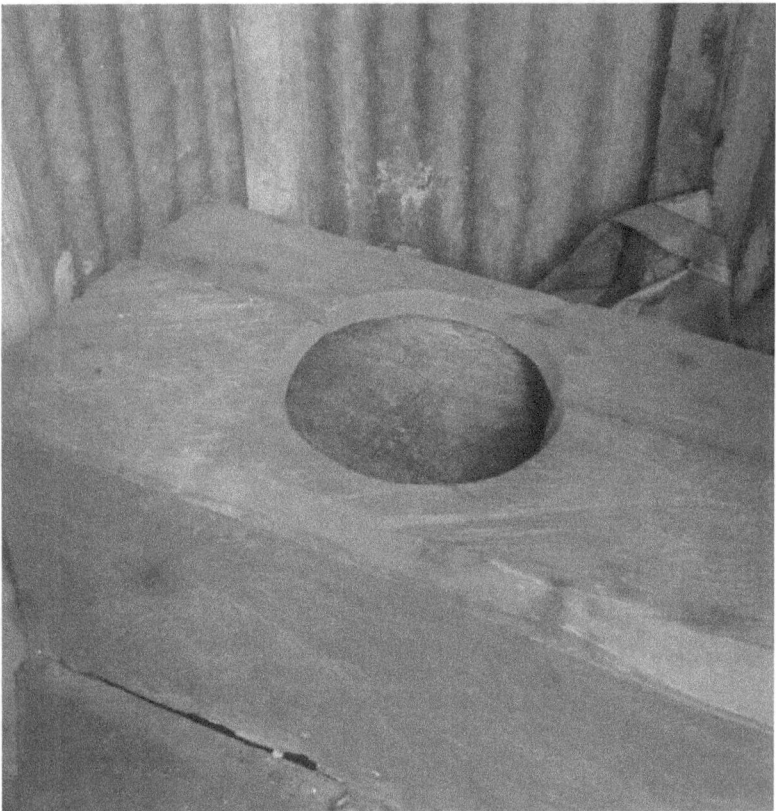

Image 10: Pit latrine.

had to describe our living conditions, and this would say how in need we were to the investigator. I remember even getting grants to purchase my books.

A so-called girlfriend of mine once cursed me saying, "You are nobody because you live in a house with a *pit toilet*," after she came to visit me one day at my childhood home. Seeing how I had lived, she tried to use it against me. It opened my eyes to the value of what a true friend is. You truly know who your friends are in your down moments. This made me more determined to succeed in my education. We have no power over where we come from, but you and I have the power to choose our own destiny guided by the hand of God Almighty. Another friend, one I grew up with in the church, told me that he did not want a friend who drove hand carts in Spanish Town.

There was a time I was messing up in university and I chose to sit out a year because I wanted to travel to America to finish my studies. This statement prompted me to get up and start moving again. Another friend said, "Shereen, I am so proud of you; you can use two ten dollars and turn it into fifty dollars." People will be people and try to put you down, but your friends will build you up. One must choose who to listen to and who to love from afar.

I shared a room with two other girls to cut down on expenses. My saved chicken money ran out and I had to think of how to feed myself and keep paying rent. On the campus, I began to sell chocolate, juice, and snacks to earn money to help pay for my basic needs. This was not new to me because as far as I can remember, I often traveled to Kingston to sell with my sisters during summer breaks to buy socks and uniform material for tuition. This setting was different for me. Now, I was among some rich and very intellectual students who never turned me away. I felt ashamed, but I was not going to give up on my goal to graduate with a BSN in nursing. With this goal at the forefront of my existence, I got through my classes. I was incredibly determined to succeed. We have to turn the negatives into positives. I was too busy to quit because I was trying to survive and get through my classes.

In my final year of nursing, my father passed away, but before he died, he got the best care ever as my colleagues and I would take turns caring for him. This feeling of satisfaction is the only payment I need to keep me going in my career. This also ensures that I give and treat every patient like my father. When you manage your own finances, you ensure that you pass the courses because if you fail, that money and time is wasted; it cannot be returned. When you are my patient, you automatically become part of my family.

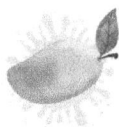

Power Thought

I had no parents to call and ask for food or rent money. There was no such thing as food stamps, shelters to spend a night, or a place to collect a breakfast in the mornings. There were no churches to go to, to get food supplies. The little I had was shared between us girls and other students who were in similar situations. God multiplied the meals that we cooked. We went to bed without eating when we did not have enough food.

Let us start showing appreciation to family and friends. When we are down, they are there. Let's cherish them in the happy times as well and build each other up. Sometimes we need to just let our hair down and listen to music and dance our crazy dance, forgetting our troubles even if it's for a minute. This is refreshing to the soul.

When you want something bad enough, you don't have any other choice but to keep moving toward it. This inner strength lies inside you and will continue to push you forward. You have the power to determine your outcome. From time to time, you may get help from other people. The important thing is to empower yourself to keep trying.

Abundant thinking looks like asking yourself what it is that you want and what it will take for you to achieve it. Whatever is in the way, remove it.

Chapter 10

The Death of My Father

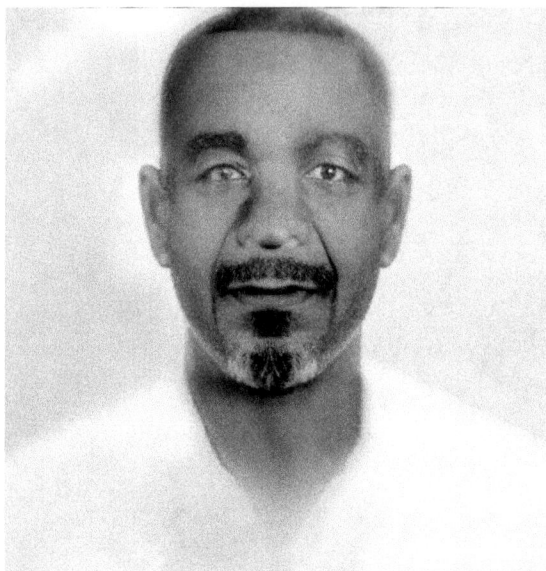

Image 11: Papa, gone but never forgotten. Father of 23 children.

y father spent nine days in hospital before passing away on June 5, 2005. Before he died, he made a few wishes known to Judith:

"Papa wanted us as sisters and brothers to take care of Mama and live as one. As he lay there knowing that he was taking his final breaths, he said these words, 'Jud mi a go dead, mi nuh have noting fi lef fi Lus, I know yuh married and soon gone. Anywhere yuh go in di world memba Mama Lus. If a one banana yuh have, mek sure she get half of it.' This he said with water pooling in his eyes [Judith, I am going to die. I have nothing to leave Lus (Mama's nickname) with. I know you are married and will soon be gone. Anywhere you go in this world, please remember your mother. If it's one banana, make sure she gets half of it.]"

This, according to Judith, was not easy. "It made me feel sad to hear someone saying this to me, that they were going to die, and I could not save them. This was not good."

When we told this to Mama, she could not believe it because she always thought that Papa did not love her. I thought, *See there—Papa did love Mama.* He also mentioned, "I want to be buried in a silver casket. I want all my daughters to carry me out of the church with Sherene at the head." I felt honored by this request because my father and I grew very close through the years. He developed diabetes combined with congestive heart failure in his last years. At the end, he fought long and hard. I was glad to be there with him as not just his daughter but also as his nurse.

He is gone. One wish that was not granted was that he wanted me to take him home to die in his bed. I refused because I did not want to give him up. In my mind, I was not ready for him to go. I can remember the early morning when, at 1:00 a.m., they called us to say that he had died. Gina and I were together at the time. I did not shed a tear because I could not believe it. Gina and I rushed to the hospital a few hours later.

"Sherene, I'm going to collect his belongings—I know it's only his clothes," said Gina.

I barely heard her as I was in denial. "Papa gone, Sherene," Gina said with tears building. I said nothing because in my mind, I was going to visit him. I expected to see my father lying on that white hospital bed with his skin nicely oiled and tanned. His eyes would be closed, but I'd be able to see equal chest expansions with his breathing. I reasoned that he was sleeping. This was how I remembered him, the last time I saw him.

When we arrived, I saw the truth. The bed was neatly spread— waiting for the next patient. There was no Papa in it. I could deny it no longer. Reality came rushing home. My tears began to flow. Gina comforted me with a hug.

"Gina, I will no longer see Papa's smiles, nor eat his chicken back. He will no longer be sitting in one of his handmade chairs, just lying there as the cool breeze sweeps over his face."

We cried together for a long time, even to the point when one of the nurses—a friend from church—came over and took me out of Gina's arms and asked, "Did they not call and told you he was gone?" Gina said, "Yes, but she did not believe." I just could not stop crying. I cried until my entire body shook. I knew death and it was the end. There is just nothing left after the person you loved and planned your life around exists no more. He was just gone, and I was not ready for him to go.

Death is just too final, too final.

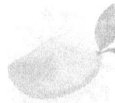

He knew God. My father got baptized in his final years on this earth in the Seventh Day Adventist church. I believe he was about seventy-three years old. His death was celebrated for two weeks as is the custom in Jamaica, The people who knew him had visited his place of residence from when he was alive, and they gathered together and played dominoes, and drank his favorite liquor, which was white rum. They shared jokes about some of the things Papa did. They shared memories of how he cared for them.

Nine-Nights

Nine-Nights is an extended wake that lasts for a few days. My father had two Nine-Nights—one at his shop for the non-Christians and the other at his home for the church community. The church members came together and sang church songs, socialized to ease the situation, and provided emotional support to the family. The non-Christian community had speakers that blasted reggae music and dance at one end. At the other end, the mannish water [goat soup] cooked over Papa's outdoor coal stove, where the orange ashes danced in the air with popping sounds and the steam twirled from the soup. Its familiar scent wafted among the mourners. I closed my eyes and Papa's image came to mind, stirring the real ram goat cooked in its herbs of scallion, thyme, scotch bonnet pepper and pimento. I exhaled a sad sigh but smiled; I could feel him with me in the aroma.

One group of people stood with liquor in hand, crying or reminiscing. On another side, a table was set up with four persons playing dominoes ['The Bones'] around it, under an improvised hanging light taken from the light pole. Their animated play added to the eclectic mix of us all grieving in our special way.

They partied that Nine-Night like my father did or would have liked. I took comfort in the fact that he was no longer suffering, and he was ready to die when it was his time. He said that last day, "My friends are all gone, am ready to go." Friends and family keep us going each day, whether we want to believe it or not, but each one of us has something that keeps us fighting. Whatever or whoever that person is, be sure to let them know."

If you've lost someone, you know how I feel and understand the words I have written. If you haven't, it is my hope that my story reminds you that you are loved.

Cherish each other as you go from day to day.

Jamaican Manish Water Recipe

Serves 5

Shared by Shelley Ann Clarke Roxborough

The quantity is based on the number of people you are going to serve.

1/2lb goat head

1/2lb goat head seed

1/2lb goat foot

1/2lb goat tripe/belly

1 cup flour

1 cup diced carrot

1 cup diced yellow yam

1 cup diced Irish potato

3 young bananas

1 cup diced cocoa (optional)

1 cup diced dasheen (optional)

8 ounces diced pumpkin

1 chocho

Spices to taste: scallion, thyme, pimento seed and pepper. Add these liberally.

Process

1. Boil goat meat till tender. Then add ground provision with dough/spinnas—rolled dumplings.
2. Add the scallion, thyme, pimento seed, and pepper. Allow to simmer until seasoned and cooked.
3. Add noodles.
4. Taste and add salt if needed.

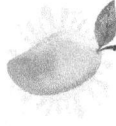

Power Thought

We are all not perfect, but in death, people fix us as such.

My father was never a perfect father. He lied to me and he cheated on Mama, but he grew to appreciate family and, most importantly, he knew who God was—he understood the true meaning of life. A man can run around all his life, but what will that profit him in the end? Some good memories, but is that enough?

What about the pain you caused others? God meets us wherever we are on this journey, and he forgives us. My mother thought my father never loved her, but from the part of him that I saw, I knew he did. She remembers only the pain he caused, and she did not visit him in his final days at the hospital. I guess this was too hard for her. We acknowledge the fact that when we hurt or wrong people, those who are hurt get to choose to give us forgiveness.

I hope I can forgive Jack one day too.

Chapter 11

Eulogy for Ivan Clarke

he events of Nine-Nights were behind us. It was time for
Papa's funeral.

Final acts, final hours, and final words reflect a life well
lived; so do the last words of our Master. When on the edge of death,
Jesus, too, got his house in order.

A final prayer of forgiveness.

A plea honored.

A request of love.

A question of suffering.

A confession of humanity.

A call of deliverance.

A Cry of Completion
(Author unknown)

"Ivan Clarke, known as Wiggy or Tawee to family and friends, began his
life on the sixth day of September 1929. Born to his late parents, Eze-
kiel Clarke and Hanna Dailey, the third of fourteen children. He grew
up in the district of Bird Mountain, Westmoreland, where he attended
Glennoily All Age school. He then continued his studies at Fare Trade
Training School, where he acquired his shoemaking skills. Later, he was
employed at Richardson's shoemaking company, where he excelled and
mastered his skills.

"Ivan's own family life began when he met Gwendolyn Thomas.
Owing to minimal employment opportunities, they later moved to
Kingston. In 1967, he was employed at the Kingston Wharf, where he

held the position of a freight handler. He later launched out as a small entrepreneur, making and repairing shoes. He was a successful business-man who managed to acquire properties and other assets. They had eight children.

"Irreconcilable differences broke him and Gwendolyn apart; how-ever, this would not hinder his search for true love. He enjoyed riding his motorbike and bicycle, and it was on his daily ride that he came across the lady who was to be his forever, Thelma Clarke. They subsequently engaged in an extensive courtship, which later resulted in marriage and the extension of his family.

"Ivan was a family-oriented person. His love and commitment for his family, has been imparted throughout his life's history. His philos-ophy on life was to live one day at a time, and to give because it is in giving that you receive. Most people will remember Ivan for his kind-ness. Although he had a shoe shop, where he repaired shoes, he also sold charcoal to people in his community and neighboring communities.

"He considered cultivation as his main hobby. The reward of this was to share with members of the community. It is also said that you were sure to get at least a cup of tea when you visited the shop. A good family man, Ivan was also an exceptional friend. Hours spent at the shop were not only for work or the provision of a warm meal he was also al-ways there to lend an ear to those in need. Counseling and the ability to incite laughter and good cheer were some of his finest qualities. He was a good motivator, especially in the lives of young people around him. He was a good husband in my eyes, a good father, and a good friend.

"In life, there are good times and bad times, good health, and ill-ness. In 1994, it was discovered that my Papa was having irregular heart-beats. He was later diagnosed with arial fibrillation. He received regular treatment at the Spanish Town Hospital; he was admitted at least twice per year for observation and treatment. God has always been good to him. Doctors, nurses, and even family members often thought that he would not make it, but doubt only served to increase his strength. You see, when God is not ready to take you home, he will mold and keep you until the time is right.

"Ivan grew up in the Baptist church and was an active member who even sang on the choir. (Yes, he had a lovely voice.) Even though he later drifted from the church, he was always spiritually minded. He eventually returned to God's truth when he became a member of the St. John's Seventh Day Adventist church in November 2004. He fought a long-dreaded illness and succumbed to this on June 5, 2005, in the Spanish Town Hospital. His last words were from a song, 'I'm waiting to hear the sweet, sweet, trumpet of the Lord.

"His last wishes were to be buried in a silver casket and for his daughters to carry him.

"He lived a full life, but most importantly, he made peace with God. He died leaving his wife Thelma Clarke, six brothers, two sisters, seventeen children, forty grandchildren, eleven great-grand, other family, and countless friends.

"The Lord will give strength unto his people. The Lord will bless his people with peace."

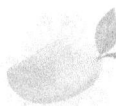

Everyone gathered after the funeral at the dead yard (the place where Papa lived before he died) for the repass. There, the family and friends fed the guests. My friends did not bother to take me home; they took me to one of their houses as I was in too much pain.

It was later passed on to me that a fight broke out between Shelly and Lorna and almost involved Gina as well. Shelly recalls:

"When Papa died, we were at the graveside. The funeral home personnel started to take him out of the hearse when Lorna and a family member of hers wanted the casket to open. I said to them, 'Let us not open it right now. Let us wait until everyone comes.' But what I think they wanted to do was to throw something in his casket. I may be wrong. Do not quote me on that one.

"Cousin Betty jumped in, 'Why yuh nuh open it' (why don't you open it)?"

'Who the hell are you,' I asked 'because I don't know you.'

'A mi aunty man' (my father's first consort's niece, which would make her Lorna's cousin).

"She started to come toward me like a fight was about to take place. Someone jumped in the middle and separated us. When Gina realized what was going on and that they wanted to fight me, she was ready to defend me. They had to pull Gina away. In that moment I felt upset because they robbed me of my tears when Papa was going down in his grave. I did not get to see or spend the last moment with him. I was too focused on bussing dem ass.

"We reached at the house for the repass. My big sister Lorna entered the gate. Mama turned to her and said, 'Mi hear weh unuh gwaan wid [I heard what was going on] at the graveside and I do not like it.'

"She started to gwaan (go on) like she wanted to shut up Mama. Her exact words were, 'Oh, it already done and gone.' And Sherene, she a come through the kitchen door or through the passage a just gave her one lick inna are forehead, mi push are inna are forehead and seh (say), 'let she talk.' And I think that was it and everyone started to separate (leave the yard). It was bad, but people grieve different ways, and years now after, it hurt so much because in the final moments, we never got to really grieve as much as we wanted to at the graveside. And then we were all hurting because it was someone we loved, gone, and this is how some people share and some people grieve, and I think this was just it."

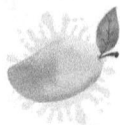

Power Thought

Love creates all kinds of emotions, and we must be tolerant of the emotions and the ways people process pain.

There will be drama in any family at any given point. This drama can escalate because of untold feelings that develop over the years that can turn into hostility.

I do believe that Lorna had a lot to say against Mama but never did. She was upset that Papa stopped seeing her mother because of my mother. To add to that, she was not happy with the way Mama treated her as her young stepdaughter. This type of tale can be confusing, especially if you were never exposed to it.

How do we as kids distance ourselves from what happened between the parents? I loved my father endlessly but resented my mother. I was upset with her for years until I learned the whole story. To move forward, take a step backward and get all the facts. I confronted Mama after gathering all the information that I could. I needed to know her reasons for not caring for Papa as I thought a wife should care for her husband, not to mention the fact that she was a Christian and should be Christlike. Now, knowing her reasons and all that she went through made me understand more, and I am now willing to forgive her. People do things, but why do they? We may see this as cruel or unfair, but what trauma occurred in that person's life to behave in such a manner? To get peace of mind, take a step backward. I am not saying what Mama did was acceptable, but it was her way of dealing with the pain she was dealt. No woman should take that kind of abuse, especially not today with so many resources at hand. Healing takes time for both the receiver and the giver. Her healing finally began with Ivan Clarke's passing.

Chapter 12

Gina Remembers

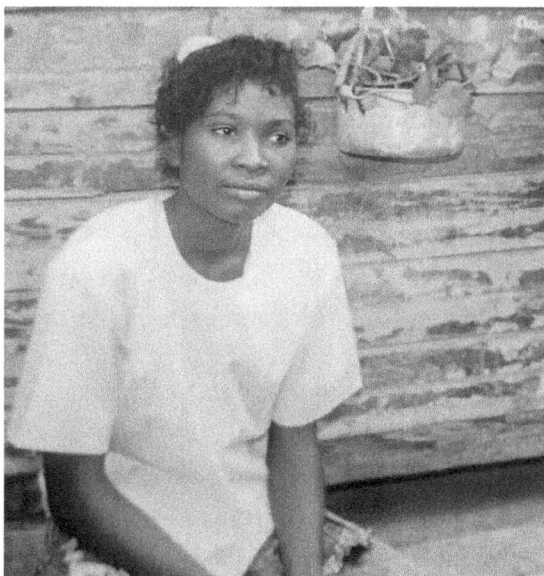

Image 12: *Gena never forgets.*

G ina, as far as you can remember, tell me about the relationship between Mama and Papa, please.

"Oh, Sherene, the history of Mama and Papa's life—Papa was a kind, hardworking person. His hands were free in giving away. He gave to the poor. Sometimes we hardly had enough in the house because a lot of times, he would go out and work and give Mama money, but a short time later he would come back for it. Whenever his children living in the state would send him clothing like pajamas or hats, he gave them away and only left himself with one. He would give most of it away."

Papa was the type of person who loved to give.

"One day he worked on a construction site. He got paid and he gave my mother ten Jamaican dollars. (In the '90s, the American dollar was roughly $8 to $10 Jamaican dollars = USD$80.) He went to Mr. Reid's shop and bought his friends liquor and paid the bills. We would sometimes purchase things on credit to survive or in order to eat from this shop. He had a friend name Mr. Bartrow, and on Friday evenings they both would drink, and sometimes he would come in drunk. He came back for the money, and when Mama would not give it to him, he box her in the face. I could not take to see my mother getting abuse. I saw her getting a lot of abuse. I could not take to see her getting hit anymore. I said to him while picking up a stone—I stepped back and yelled 'I will burst your head!' He said to me 'You a woman now?' He ran me down toward The Commons, but he could not catch me. I said to him again, 'If you touch my mother again, I am going to burst your head!' He threw out my clothes, all of them, outside, including my machine that Judith buy me to do fashion designing."

Gina was clearly upset at this memory. "Take your time, Gina."

"After everything simma (cool down), he was all right again. He called me one day and told me to stay in the shop, he is going to the market to buy yam. A lady came by when he was gone. She asked, 'Mr. Ivan is not here?' I said to her, 'No.' She said she came to buy two pan of coal (charcoal) and she not paying is come she com to trus (credit). I told her no. After Papa come back, I told him this and he said nothing. Another day now, and Mama was not there, the same lady came back through the back gate to my father. She lived in Ebony (this was a housing scheme beside us—a community built up with concrete structures, what we would call a residential area in the United States). I started thinking that this woman is always coming for free things. You know, I start to understand big people story now. So, I started to put things together now and I told her not to come back here, or else I will chop her up with my machete because she is robbing what we suppose to get. She was robbing our father money. And I tell you something, she go and tell Papa. Papa came home and said, 'Gina, a lady came for coal, and you told her you are going to chop her up.' I told him, 'I do not know anything about this.'

Looking back on this memory, it seems very funny to me. We let our words get the better of us sometimes. Sherene, I do not know how am still alive. I got so mad (angry), my father work a lot of money and sometimes he had none because of those women. I got really bringle (angry) with Papa.

"I don't know why am still alive. I would even fight with Taddy (our brother). He would cook and not share with us. I just fight with him. As I got older, I started to understand what was going on. I started looking out for my mother and sisters and brothers. I get to understand that him love woman and is wild and love to fight my mother and disrespect her, saying she have man, a church, and all that. Hey, Sherene, you see Mama. She lived a rough life with Papa, a really rough, rough life. When I was small, he would cuss (argue) her and raise his voice after her. She went through a lot of that. I use (past tense) to pre (study) him, and I would often say to myself, 'I cannot wait until I get big.' That's the reason why Mama never loved Papa in the last part of his life.

"As I grew older, one day, he came in to fight Mama and he hit her in her face. I got so angry, but I could not do nothing because I was too small.

"Do you know what Mama said? She said she was going to leave and go to sister Walton and live (mother did days' work with this church lady). That made me so angry because my mother not leaving me. But Sherene, I believed that Mama did genuinely love Papa, but after all that abuse, she did not return the feelings. This abuse happened since I was three years old. My father made sure that we eat and have a roof over our heads, but he did not care about school. All he cared about was the road.

"My father was a hell from a long time, and he loved woman. He cared enough for us to eat food. In growing up, my mother was never happy. Her happy days are now, after he is dead and gone. He would go in the room and lock the door and use him strength on her and friend her up. Mama would often sleep with us, and he would come for her. Sometimes, Sherene, he would say 'Yuh nah come inna di bed, yuh nah come inna di bed (you are not coming in the bed)', and he would draw her into the room. From I am small, I use to be sorry for my mother.

Hey, Sherene, I do not like remembering these things cause water come a mi (my) eyes to see what my mother went through. It's because you all don't know enuh. Mama did not live a normal life. That is why today I don't take talk from no one. You see Mama her life when she a grow us was not a happy one, and then Lorna (sister from my father side) and her mother and other people that tried to fight her out and same time she a think on them and think on us, was not pretty for her."

"When did she get baptized?" I asked.

"This is not so clear on my side, but after she is looking for help, a way of serving God, she did not see another way out. She went to the Spanish Town church and got baptized. There was a lady called Miss Jackson. She would come and visit and carry clothing and shoes so Mama could put on clothe to go to church.

"This lady who was a colporteur became close friend with Mama. She told Papa and he said, 'Him not going to church to do no wickedness.' She had to change church to St. John's as this was closer to us. She could not manage to take all of us to church in Spanish Town as this was too far.

"After a while we had to move because the people wanted their land we lived on. He found a piece of land near to his brother and that's where we grew up. Mama steadfast in her church and my father did not believe he should go to church. It was after he got sick then he decided to get baptized. Her friend sis Jackson was awesome. Friday evening time we use to go for clothe and food from her. We did not even have panty or if we did, they would be too big, and we would tie it at the sides. On Sabbath we could hardly find food. She would buy a box of oats with milk from what he gave her for Sabbath lunch. Sometimes no change was left, and he would come back for the money. This made me mad. Until after a while him stop work and he would go into the field and come back with mango and cane (sugar cane), and we would eat so-so mango and go to bed. You all do not remember, but our bringing up was not nice. It was rough.

"You see, Marie use to bawl (cry) all the time, she hungry. Nothing for her to eat. She was small. We used to say she was bawli bawli (cry cry), but she hungry. She will be crying but she is not saying anything.

As I get older and understand, I realized that is hungry; my sister was hungry. Even today, if nothing happens to Marie, she will not talk; she will hold it. She used to bawl (cry) until Mama come home.

"A cannot talk anymore. It is too much for me to remember. Growing up, nothing pretty, Marie bawl (cry), Shelly asthma tek har (Shelly would have an asthma attack). Mama had no money to take her to hospital and this woman would boil up bush and give my sister to drink. This made her worst and made her have rotten teeth (tooth decay). Every day I talk, I don't know how my sister is still living."

Gina started to cry.

"Sometimes Judith, our eldest sister," she sniffles "and she married to an abusive man, and sometimes we use to see Judith like once a month. Sometimes she would carry things for me. The shorts that you see in the picture, Judith bought that shorts for me. Everywhere I go a wear it.

"She sent me to fashion school and that blouse I sew and wear it with that shorts. I saw her another long time and I had no shoes on my feet and there was this old one. I put it on, and she said she was going to buy me a shoe as that one was in a bad condition. The following week she did not buy it because something went wrong with her toilette paper business but the following, she buy it.

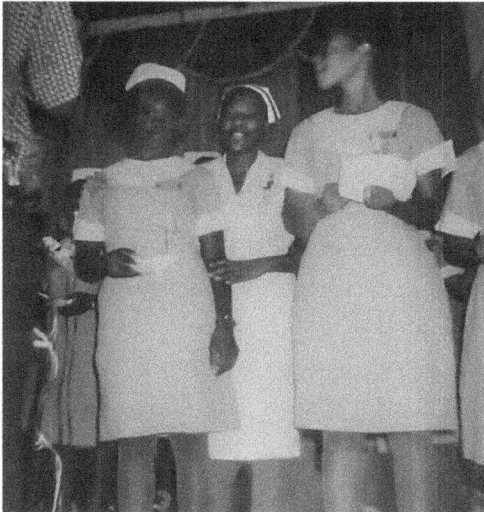

Image 13: Nursing students capping ceremony (2002). I'm the nurse on the left.

"She bought me the shoes, it's the best my foot ever feels. I get a pair a new shoe to wear on my feet. I learned later that her husband was beating her, and she moved and lived close beside us and even then, she had to run up and down from Jim Brown (her husband's name). The only thing I can say is I thank God we alive today and we can eat and we can drink, but back in the days—eighteen years old, fifteen, sixteen, fourteen, thirteen, twelve, eleven, ten, nine, eight, seven, six, five, four—were not pretty ones."

All because Gina refused to return to the life we had growing up. It was a nightmare to her, and for all of us to some extent. We know the value of working together. We are not perfect, but for the most part, us six girls who experienced this with our parents keep looking out for one other.

Sometimes this scares me because we are close, and at times we hurt each other, but through it all, if one hurts, we all hurt.

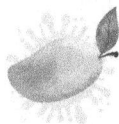

Power Thought

As parents, we need to realize that what we do affects our kid directly or indirectly. How Papa treated Mama left us, his children, thinking that this is acceptable behavior in marriage. Grown up, we will come to accept the same treatment from men or become insecure about relationships.

What does our instinct tell us about a relationship that we are in? Are you hearing that small voice that says something is just not right or adding up? Sometimes we need to listen to the voice of God. Believe it or not, he speaks to us.

What do we do with the part of us that we consider to be no good? We need to own ourselves and say if this part of us is holding us back, correct it, let it go, and walk away with the positive. Use it to build you into a stronger human being.

Part Two

Mixed Review: Jamaican Dating Mindset

Chapter 13

Hanging Out

Two famous terms used when I was younger in Jamaica when dating are "wi-huck-up" or "wi-link-up." The "wi-huck-up" is more of an American term and means that two individuals become sexually intimate before getting to know one another well. It is during this type of encounter that they learn about the other partner. If a man gives a woman a gift of lingerie or undergarments, it is his way of testing to see if you are willing to be intimate with him. If you accept the gift, it sends the message that yes, you like him enough to move forward with him. If you reject the gift, it sends a message that he has to work harder, with the possibility of never getting to the next level.

This seemed backward and that it should not be the case for me as a Christian girl. I felt too much guilt to consider doing something outside of marriage, even though it was widely accepted and practiced by the young people in the church. The adults knew that the young ones practiced this and made a huge effort to push early marriage. These early marriages usually ended in divorce after two or three years. Otherwise, the "link-up-end-up-mash-up" is the breakup that might occur after a few weeks with the unmarried ones.

The wi-link-up is where we get together as a group and go to the movies, the mall, or church. It's not really dating but a good way to socialize. In the Jamaican culture, wi-link-up more than wi-huck-up.

My nephew Tyrese is twenty-one years old. He loves that he can date anyone in Florida. When he visited Jamaica, he felt that the women were more opportunistic because he speaks with an American accent. He thinks that the difference between Jamaican and American women is that the islanders respect their parents and the Americans are more casual about respect. He also thinks that if he was to live in Jamaica, he could possibly find someone who would love him for who he is. To him, Jamaican women seem to be more focused and know what they want. He appreciates women who have goals and can think ahead ten years instead of live in the moment, just for fun. Regardless of our culture or early dating experiences, this first season impacts the way we see ourselves the rest of our lives. Rejection can impact self esteem, and bad decisions may lead to shame. This is not a season to discount as frivolous, as it is a defining time in every human life. We all want to love and be loved and, feel accepted, and we desire others to notice us. Navigating these dating years can be confusing.

I want to be a role model for Nathan and teach him how to respect his parents and how to treat women. I teach him how, as a man, he has to be aware of keeping the house safe, support the household chores, and learn how to buy gifts without a hidden agenda, except for my birthday. When it comes time for him to date, he will know how to respect and treat a woman right. With dating in the Seventh Day Adventist church community, we girls are looked down upon by the older sisters when we date because they assume that we are throwing ourselves at and sleeping with everyone. This is not true. Dating is not about having one partner or sleeping with each other. It is about going out in groups with several people and getting to know more about the opposite sex in a safe environment. We will naturally improve our dating skills as well as learn how to socialize. This group process helps us to know how to go about choosing one compatible life partner, the right person. In our church, we tended to be pressured into marriage by a certain age in order to have children. It was only acceptable in the church to have children within wedlock. While this is true, it put us at risk of rushing into marriage to the wrong person, which often caused an increase in the divorce rate, even in the church.

I had my first boyfriend at the age of twenty-one. It was not really a boyfriend/girlfriend kind of thing. I just wanted to test the waters. The thing with Jamaican men is that if you go out on a date with them, they do not expect you to sleep with them, especially if they want a serious relationship. If you did succumb to their advances, they'd consider you cheap. This same double standard exists in the American culture, yet it appears to be a normal expectation that you sleep with each other on the first date.

In this way, Jamaican men feel more respectful.

I was wearing a floral miniskirt and walking along a street in Portmore when I met my first boyfriend. He was fixing his car, and as I passed, he said hello. I did not answer him, but I subconsciously slowed my walk. He took notice and left his car to run after me.

"Hi," he said.

"Why did you run after me?" I asked.

"Because I saw that you slowed your pace."

Hmmmm, eye for details! I thought to myself. I liked how he looked—very muscular, clean white teeth, and nice lips. What girl does not love a man with nice lips and a clean mouth?

"I would like to cook you dinner at my house in Kingston. Will you come?" he asked.

I wanted to see what this sex thing was like. I was not looking for a boyfriend at the time. I decided I would go. I planned to break the rules and sleep with this guy on the first date. I was tired of not knowing. I am twenty-one years old. Am ready. I reasoned with myself.

"Yes, I will join you for dinner."

He indeed cooked me dinner. I was tired of being a virgin and just afraid of having sex because I did not want to get pregnant. In the Jamaican culture, an unplanned pregnancy almost always impacted the future of the mother. She was expected to keep her child and care for it. It was a sure bet that she would be lowly educated and work menial tasks the rest of her life. My idea was to get an education and upgrade myself from the cultural thinking. A baby for me was out of the question. But here, flirting with this man, my double-mindedness could threaten my future plans.

It was my first sexual encounter, and our intimate relationship ended after two months when he migrated to the United States. Looking back at this relationship, I must admit that I was disappointed. I gave up my virginity too easily after keeping it so long. I held out so long, not only for the fear of pregnancy but for spiritual reasons. I did enjoy myself in the moment. Afterward, the guilt began to seep into my soul.

During my dating period, I went to the movies to "get-to-know-each-other," which looked like the two of us visiting one another's homes. This ideal setup for sexual opportunities eventually got to me because I always felt guilty knowing that we were not married. I heard about fornication and adultery in the church through sermons. The emphasis was always about purity. The message was reinforced by Mama because she did not want me to make the same mistake she had.

I did know better. But I also had the example of my father's relationship with my mother, even though her thinking had transformed since her baptism in the church. Hers was not a healthy relationship. As a child witness to my own family dynamics, how could I possibly know what to accept throughout the dating period, even though I heard in church not to do it? The messages were confusing. It is important as parents to set good examples for our sons and daughters to emulate.

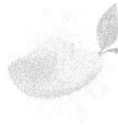

What is dating really? My God sister (godmother) Tashel and I discussed our Jamaican dating experiences and compared notes. I found it interesting how different our experiences were, even though we belonged to the same Seventh Day Adventist church congregation.

"Tashel, what was your dating experience in Jamaica?"

"Sherene, I am thirty-eight years old and did not have the cliché dating experience growing up in the church that I have now, where we group date. Back then, it was the rule of the household that I was not allowed to have a boyfriend until was twenty-one years old. So, you know that going out on a date was not entertained. At the age of fourteen, I had friends; one was Kirkland.

"Was Kirkland your boyfriend?"

"No, we were not in an intimate relationship with one another, we just hung out. He was eighteen years old, and I eventually hid it from my grandmother and dated him. We did drive around in Kingston and Spanish Town, but the one notable thing about that relationship is that he opened and closed the car door for me. He treated me like a lady. I got use to this and when I was around other males, I knew that they should be opening and closing doors. My family did not know that I was going out with men of the opposite sex."

"Tashel, did your grandmother ever find out?"

"No. My first open relationship was London. I liked him very much. As a boyfriend London was sweet. He would buy me little gifts. I like chocolate. Every time I saw him, he would buy me chocolate—milky chocolate. He would put the chocolate in his mouth and tell me to come get it. That is where the kissing began. We were never sexually intimate, but we petted and kissed. My body was going through so many different changes by the time I was fourteen years old. I had no adults I felt comfortable with enough to talk about these changes, so I spoke with my friends who were sexually active. The relationship with London did not last long as he cheated on me with another woman at the church who was involved in another relationship. At that age I did not know how to handle this, and I was overly aggressive toward the girl and to London."

We both laughed about how silly and naive we were.

"Years down the line, we talked about our relationship for closure and I asked him why he hurt me like that. He said that my grandma played a role in this because she did not like him, and we could not do anything beyond seeing each other at church. He claimed his friends in sixth form were older and advised him that I was way too young to even go into a movie theater with or go out on group dates with them. They also informed him that he was robbing the cradle. London said, and I quote, 'Tashel, you may be a nice person, but you are too young to be in a committed relationship with one person.'"

"Why did your mama (grandmother) not like him?"

"There was a big age difference. I was fourteen in fourth form and he was eighteen. At that age, it was different because we could not go to a restaurant together. Even though Mama knew about it, she did not approve because London was from an abusive household, and she feared that I might become a part of that cycle. She did not see that life for me, but London and I fooled around with each other for years."

"How did your mama deal with that?"

"My grandmother feared I would become a teenage mother like my mom. She would take me to the doctor in Spanish Town every year from twelve years old to sixteen to check and see if I was still a virgin. She stopped at sixteen because the doctor told her not to bring me back as it was child abuse."

I laughed.

"Why are you laughing?" Tashel asked, chuckling.

"Because checking to see if you are a virgin does not stop anything from happening."

"She was crazy or just overprotective, but in spite of the experience, it made me very afraid of getting pregnant."

"Okay, so your grandmother put the fear of God in you—just like my mama—so what happened next?"

"Let me tell you about the bet. London's best friend, Marcos, dated London's sister, but they broke up. We were all part of the Pathfinder Club at church. Marcos had the bright idea while walking home from a meeting one night to confess his feelings to me. He told me he liked me very much, his friend London is an idiot, and that they had a bet to see who could have sex with me first to break my virginity. Marcos and I were never in a relationship or talked about having feelings for each other. This really hurt my feelings. At that age, I felt that there was no genuine love or respect for me as a woman. Everyone knew that I loved London, and that was a learning experience for me. Not having anyone to talk to about this was difficult. I had all these feelings to figure out and then finding out about this bet was like the ultimate feeling of betrayal. It really affected my self-worth.

"Fast forward to the age of sixteen, when I met Keino. At 4:30 a.m. every morning, I had to get a taxi to go to school in Kingston, which was a half an hour drive. The island traffic could take up to three hours. Every morning, this family would honk their horn as they passed by me. I could tell that they thought it was a funny thing to do. This went on for months. One day, we were coming home from a sixth form concert on a rainy Friday night. My hair was wet and very thick. My hair elastic had burst, and my hair came loose and turned into an afro puff. The place was full of people and the extra-long bus was packed. I immediately recognized the guy from the honking car and noticed he was kind of cute. I was with my friends Natalie, Michelin, and a whole group of Kingston College (KC) boys. We all knew one another by our uniforms. I was the quiet one, always insecure about my looks, so all my friends were engaged in conversation (except for me) with the KC boys. I stood there just watching and laughing nervously. Then there comes Mr. Keino— the honker. At the time, I did not know his name, but we called him the guy with the dimples. He had some beautiful dimples too—they were real pretty! He caught the eyes of Michelin and, of course, mine. Michelin was engaged with the other guys from Kingston College and broke to whisper in my ears, 'I like the guy with the dimples, and I want his number—can you write him a letter for me?' I was the writer in the group, so I agreed. I found a folder leaf in my bag and began to write a secret admirer letter for Michelin. Ah, I wrote him the sweetest admirer letter ever. Lord have mercy on my soul," she laughed. "It read:

"Roses are red, violets are blue,
You have the sweetest dimples,
And a secret admirer. Can you guess who?
Respond with your number at the bottom of the paper."

"I was very sharp," she laughed.

"He did not respond but he blushed instead. A lady on the bus saw what was going on and said, 'Why did you do this to the poor young man—you have him blushing in public!' He did not respond. At that time, we felt that the note was a flop because of his silent blushing.

"Michelin was okay because she still had the attention of one of those cute, Chinese-looking Kingston College boys. I could not stop looking at him. I thought he was so handsome."

"What happened next?"

"When he got off the bus, he waited for me, walked over, and said, "I am not interested in the person who asked you to write the note. I heard everything she asked you to do because the bus was so packed. I am interested in the person who wrote the note."

I asked, "Why?"

'That person has a soul,' he said.

He gave me his number and asked me to call him after church. He knew it was me."

"Did you call him, Tashel?" I asked.

"Girl, that was the first Adventist Youth program I missed! There was no Mama around, she was at church, thank God. She was *not* going to mess up my plans. We were on the phone from 3 p.m. to 8 p.m. just talking. The next weekend, I learned that he had already told his mother about me. One day I walked to the bus stop on my way from school and standing there, waiting, was Keino."

"Keino, why are you here?"

"I am waiting for you, Tashel."

"I never forgot that; it was so sweet. His mom came and picked us up and dropped me off at home. We rode in the back of their van just laughing and talking. That, for me, was significant, and I will tell you why—it made me feel special. For him to come to my bus stop from where his school was, he had to take a bus in the opposite direction from school to meet me. So, he had thought about what he was doing before he did it. That is why I felt special."

"When did you start dating each other?"

"This was part of my dating experience. From their (guys) actions, I understand how they felt about me—not just by words alone. All the time before this experience, it was me trying to navigate what dating was and understanding people of the opposite sex based on their actions. For me, it was the feeling I got based on their actions. I will tell you what he did—he always looked out for me to make sure that I was okay. He was certainly a protector."

"How did he protect you?" I asked.

"Buses were always going on strike. I can remember on one such occasion, Keino and twelve of his friends came to the Crossroad bus stop where I waited for my bus. I was literally stranded. They knew a taxi driver and all twelve boys chartered him. They all came together to pay the taxi driver for me to get home!"

"That sounds crazy!"

"It *was* crazy. Can you imagine, Sherene, one girl with twelve boys in a taxi? It was the hunch-back taxi, too! When we got to Spanish Town, his parents picked me up and took me home."

"On Sabbath evenings, it was movie night at his house. His mom would pick the movie. I did not have cable, so I did not know about movies. She would have the boys do their thing and sit outside and watch television. She would invite me to lie on her bed and watch movies and have girl talk.

"One day he came to my house, and I did not know he was coming. He wanted me to spend time with his family. He asked my grandmother's permission for his family to come and get me. He spoke to my aunt and met my whole family without my knowledge. Isn't that interesting? And my grandmother told him he was a respectable young man and told him it was okay.

"That was the beginning of my dating experience with him. Isn't that something? With that experience, all that I learned about dating came through his family. We had game night and movie night and were never allowed to be alone. He made sure I felt comfortable and protected, and he always told me that I was beautiful. We studied, prayed together, and tried to build our future years together. He planned to be a doctor and I was going to be the lawyer. He taught me what unconditional love was and did not care that I was poorer than him. He taught me that my life was not the situation that I was born with but what I choose to do with this life I was given."

"Every time I think about his mother, I get sad because I felt lost without him and his family. After he died, I did not know who I was without him. He gave me a feeling that I belonged. I never slept with Keino, and we were both virgins."

Keino died tragically trying to rescue a friend from drowning.

Another time I spoke with Sondra about her dating experience in Jamaica.

"Delpha, it was good. I will not lie. When you go out with a guy, you do not have to worry about who will pay the meal or whether or not he would ask for sex at the end of the first or second date. Bear in mind, Jamaican men believe that if a woman sleeps with them on the first date, she is no good. In terms of when you enter into a relationship, it is a given that he will keep you financially and sexually secure."

"What do you mean by that?"

"When you live in the home, he knows how to pay the bills. And he knows how to take care of you financially. The only problem is that they believe, I will be frank, 'one pussy kill cocky' (laugh), so be prepared for either leaving or having an STD at some point in the relationship."

"How did you handle this infidelity, if that happened to you?"

"Well, it happened to me when I was pregnant with my daughter,
and I put him out. I took him back, but a cheater will always be a cheater. I am better for leaving."

"Romance wise, how was that part of it?"

"The romance was good because if a guy likes you, it would be good. He would tell you—and its much like that with the guy I am dating now, he is like that too—you do not have to wonder where you stand and so on."

"Sondra, is he a Jamaican?"

"No. He is a Caucasian. I said I cannot take the cheating. This does not mean that Caucasian men don't cheat. But I took my time picking him. Some women will disagree and don't mind as long as they are fi-nancially secure. But I can tell you from personal experience, having a woman come to your house to curse you about your man who lives with you is not a nice feeling. All that coupled with the emotional distress, with the fear of contracting a non-curable STD that might lead to death, is not a cup from which anyone should drink. I prefer to have a relation-ship and work to achieve my financial objectives and have my partner be faithful emotionally, physically, and mentally to me than to have all the money in the world and have a son of a bitch that cheats all the time."

"You said you took your time to pick him. Explain?"

"When I just started talking to him, I was not very welcoming emo-tionally, and I told him all my bad traits or character upfront. And he stuck around. I did not pretend. I wanted him to see the worst of me. He hung around, now he is seeing the best of me."

"I want you to compare the dating scene here, now living in Amer-ica, with how you the see Jamaica dating?"

"Totally different. With that in mind, there is no absolute. Dating here [in the US] you will go on the first date and they expect to sleep with you, and that is quite normal. They will want to sleep with you and will do it if you let them, and for years, without once asking if you have soap to wash your private parts. Now this is from a woman who says finances is not everything, but coming from a Jamaican background, where a man knows what he is supposed to do in terms of finances, that was a real culture shock. The men here are also very fragile. They want you to always say that they are king, but God forbid if you should raise your voice at them or say anything against their manly traits; then they shrivel."

"Do they carry you out on dates?"

"Yes, they carry you out on dates, but the dates here are never just going out to know someone. It is usually about getting through the date to get to the sexual encounter. Once again, no absolute. I was lucky, yes, to meet someone who was willing to get to know me before wanting sexual intimacy. Whether or not the relationship lasts, whether there is infidelity, whether there is financial support, emotional distress, or fulfillment, each individual must decide what they are worth. And once again, I can't take the cheating."

This misguided cultural mindset is hardly wholesome. Parents, train your children right and take your children out on dates. Traditional dating, where the parents meet the guy or girl you are going out with, sounded ancient to us growing up, which is why it was not really practiced in the cultural norms of Jamaican society. I have discovered that the wi-huck-up gets you nowhere, is full of strife, contains no lifetime of joy, and is all for something temporary. I am no longer interested in that behavior, and I'm reluctant to use the terms in this book but felt it necessary to share the reality of the cultural norms. At the end of the day, we must teach ourselves self-respect.

Fathers have an opportunity to teach their girls growing up how they should be taken out on dates. This will teach them to know how to be treated. In this process, the father will take his daughter out, open the car door for her, and let her get comfortable.

When seated in a restaurant, he will pull her chair out for her to sit, pay for her meal, and have meaningful discussions. In doing this, a standard is set, and the young lady will know what to expect. The sons will also try to emulate this standard set by the father. Mothers should do the same and teach their sons how to cherish and treat them with respect. When this is not taught, how can one know what is proper versus what is not? Everywhere I look, the youth today are left lacking in this department because they were not taught properly. I was not taught that by my father.

I love to imagine what it might have been like if my father and mother had done this for our family. I forgive them because they did not know any different. My father showed his love and respect for me in other ways by trying to provide for us as best he could and taught us to love each other. He did not go beyond the basic needs because he did not know something else existed. He just did what he knew to do. For that, I love him. I also love that I knew him because he was present.

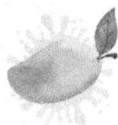

Power Thought

I was in a place where I wanted to explore the world and experience something that was not under the all-consuming influence of church. I wanted more than what the church taught. I wanted to know what was "out there" for myself. God was with me and I knew it, but he was not the center of my world then. I knew he was with me because I was never content when I did the things God was not pleased with. The small voice kept whispering to me, *Come home.* No matter how far away you try to run from God, just know you cannot outrun him. When you are his, you are *his only*, and he has your back until you find your way back home.

When we come back to God, we may have some lifetime consequences from the ungodly decisions we made when we strayed, but for those who believe in him, God will use all those experiences to glorify him. We become the teachers who can inspire others. Later, when I got married and lived in the Turks and Caicos Islands, I was even more convicted about the Jamaican wi-link-up influences in the culture. I wanted to impact the younger generation about doing things in a way that was more pleasing to God.

As a youth leader in a Turks and Caicos church, years after I was married and all my rebellion was behind me. I was asked to educate the church members about dating, and to define the term 'dating' to the elderly population in particular because in their minds, the youth were wild, meaning that they were having more than one intimate relationship and should not be having sex.

Most people are of the belief that dating is having one exclusive partner. I even believed this before I taught that program. Now that I knew what the consequences were with my own poor decisions, I wanted to help the youth understand what dating is and choose a better way to behave because some consequences are for life.

I taught them about the benefits of group dating. The elders were more receptive of the group dating scenario I presented, as were the youth because they wanted the church to understand and not judge them. I am very happy with the outcome of our meeting because the adults understood that they had to stop acting sanctimoniously with the youth. The youth learned that there were better ways to get to know one another, such as group dating. Everyone came away with a better understanding.

Believe in the beauty of you. The uniqueness that you bring to a relationship might just be the reason that your partner falls in love with you. Love the "crazy" you first, then others will gravitate to the beauty they see in you as they cherish and respect you.

Chapter 14

The Influence of Adorable Yohan

Before I came back to God, I formed a relationship with Yohan that I attribute to giving me a huge step out of poverty. I was a very naïve twenty-six-year-old. He was my psychology professor in nursing school.

One day in class, my group discussed our Rastafarianism project. I shared with a group member my experience interviewing a Rasta man in person. In my mind, who better to discuss their customs and beliefs than them? I searched for one. As I stepped through the gates of the university in my nursing uniform, I saw a Rasta man sitting on the corner.

"Hello, my name is Delpha. I'm a nursing student and I have a class project where we are studying Rastafarianism, and I'm wondering if you might be interested in coming to speak to our class about your beliefs?" Eventually, I convinced him to come as a guest speaker.

"Okay, I will be your guest."

Looking back, I could not believe I was able speak to a stranger and coordinate this. I, Delpha, the girl who had little confidence, talked him into coming to do an interview with me in front of a room full of college students. The experience gave me hope for myself and abilities.

Yohan saw my lack of confidence and often reminded me to believe in myself. He tried to teach me how to appreciate myself for who I was and shared how much he saw of my potential because I was a woman of action. Even though it is true, I struggled to believe in myself.

I knew Yohan liked me because of the way he looked at and spoke to me. I could feel his eyes on me whenever I walked away. Our relationship started after I graduated from nursing school. I found him to be such a charismatic person to talk with, and he was so full of knowledge and was well-spoken and well respected.

The first time Yohan came to visit me, one Sunday evening at my board house in Frazer Content, I was impressed by his humility. He came to my poor little abode, removed his shoes at the door, and sat in the only chair in the room while I sat at his feet. We had a wonderful conversation about a recent trip he had just come home from, and he'd bought me something. He smiled as he handed me a simple white gift bag.

I peeked inside, smiling, and could see it was a green bathing suit.

"Thank you, Yohan, I love it!" My smile would not quit as I blushed.

He did not expect me to sleep with him; that I am sure of because of how we spoke to each other at school—with respect.

He showed me how a man was to treat a woman during the time we were together; he taught me about life, money management, business, and success principles for life. I do believe that God sends someone to be in your life at the time you need that person. He paid for everything I needed, and he taught me how to pay off my student loan. He gave me his old car to drive when he bought a new one and invested in my new business of selling nursing supplies.

I asked him later, "What made you choose me?"

"I liked how you looked; you have a nice shape."

Okay! Why is it that men initially go after women based on how they look?

"Later, I saw where you were coming from and saw how you lived. I noticed how incredibly determined you are."

He shared his version of how to run a household in a committed relationship. I fell in love with Yohan.

Women do not usually accept personal gifts like this if they are not interested. At the time, I did not know he was testing me to see if I was just as interested in him as he was in me. He knew that when I accepted this gift that I would move forward with him. My faith was still in development and not as strong as it is now in the church.

We attended plays or went to dinner. I admired his intellect. We had a wonderful connection. Financially, he purchased everything I needed in the house. Responsible Jamaican men were known to take care of their women in this way. He encouraged me to concentrate on paying off my student loan while he took care of everything else in the house. Every coin I earned in the next six months went toward the loan. He taught me to purchase things with cash and avoid credit. He reinforced what my mother taught me regarding money management. This was the beginning of my journey toward breaking free of my poverty mindset.

My new business selling nursing uniforms required a van, so I purchased a van with a down payment. Yohan invested 100,000 Jamaican dollars in the license and insurance for one year. I paid the rest of the van loan off with the earnings from the business. I had it good with Yohan in certain aspects. Compared to him, I felt unequal and that I had to prove myself. I had to show that I was faithful, a woman worthy of him. He certainly did not put himself on a pedestal, but I was in awe and held a great amount of respect for him. I gave Yohan no reason to doubt my loyalty, but he did because I had two male friends I would not give up. These church friends were from my childhood, the ones who lived in better communities and houses than myself.

Once I drove his car in a particular neighborhood to get something done with a girlfriend. One of his friends told him about seeing the car there and Yohan believed that I went to see a man. This was not true, but that one little doubt put a strain on our relationship. Our eighteen-year age difference was also an issue. I was not as mature as he was. He expected a lot of things from me that I was not able to handle due to my lack of life experience. He felt I should have been better able to handle some situations. The truth is, I was just not there yet.

I successfully graduated from nursing school in 2005. I did not feel the exhilaration that I should have with the graduation experience because Papa was not there to celebrate my success with me. I just focused on work to make money and pay off my school debt. I worked overtime to repay the Student Loan Bureau for my debt. Perhaps this was a distraction for the grief I felt with the passing of Papa, but it was a good one. With the help of Yohan, I was able to pay it off in six months and experience the exhilaration of being debt free. Graduation was more of a major milestone to celebrate because it was a huge step toward getting out of poverty. There are students like me who still need financial assistance. I knew that if I could quickly pay back what was loaned to me, others could have the same opportunity awarded to them.

Years later, Yohan and I talked. He revealed, in hindsight, that he was insecure because of our age difference. I found this to be upsetting news and felt insecure in response. I realized Yohan did love me much more than I knew. I missed his brilliance and intelligence. Today, I am incredibly grateful for what he taught me.

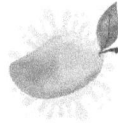

Power Thought

Explore your surroundings. Find joy and happiness in the little blessings God has given you. Make your life meaningful to you. Give when you can or when you are financially stable enough before extending a helping hand to others. In other words, give wisely.

Yohan helped me financially and emotionally; he made me believe more in myself and my dreams. I came to appreciate help more in this stage of my life. People pass through your life for a reason. Some were meant to stay while others were sent to teach you a lesson. Embrace those lessons and make the change.

Chapter 15

Could Jamaica Really Afford Free Healthcare?

In April 2008, Prime Minister Orette Bruce Golding made healthcare free in Jamaica. This was promised during his election campaign and was one reason why he won the election. He kept his promise. With this new free healthcare, more patients began to utilize the healthcare system. Resources ran shorter than they had already been. The "free" system was worse than before. Nurses and doctors were overworked. The medical equipment was falling apart and wasn't maintained or replaced in a timely manner. In the end, patients had to pay out of pocket to get a CT scan done. In the hospital where I worked, the CT scanner broke down. People got frustrated over the long hours of wait time that they had to experience. Some who could afford it turned to private hospitals and doctors' offices. The question then is, who was healthcare really free to or for? It was a mess.

I felt the impact of this so-called free healthcare. I worked for three years in Jamaica as a registered nurse, one of which I spent working on the medical-surgical unit at a private hospital. Yet, I was restless and felt like I needed more than just a routine job in Jamaica. I decided to work in emergency nursing. I moved on to the University Hospital of the West Indies, where I worked for six months to become certified in emergency nursing in the emergency room. I loved the fast pace of the ER and thrived in the organized chaos. During my training, I realized that the ER was a great fit for me. It felt good to know that I'd made the right decision. Fifteen years later, I still work as an emergency room nurse because I love it so much.

While working in the ER, sometimes we did not have adequate supplies. We often used cardboard to make soft collars for people with suspected spinal cord injuries. We did not have the famous Aspen C-collar (a neck brace) very often. We had our makeshift collar cut out to mimic the shape of the neck. We would then wrap it in stockinet and place it around the neck for support. Other resources were sometimes short too, and we had to improvise. I was often doing day duty and the ER would be filled up with patients, yet when the eight hours shift was at an end, the department was still filled with patients. This made me feel useless. Nurses had to take their own patients out of the department to have their CAT scan or X-rays done. Upon arrival in the sonography department, it would be full, and you had to wait. This caused a backup of patients being seen in the ER. This third world system was not properly organized, and there was nowhere to voice concerns without being classified as a fault finder. It was just overbearing to me, and I had to get out before I lost my sanity.

My friend Alicia took her ten-year-old son, Raheim, to the ER in Jamaica for his acute myeloid leukemia, and we talked about her experience.

"Alicia, while Raheim was being admitted to the hospital, were you there with him?"

"Yes, I was there with him for one month, but then I had to leave Jamaica and return to the Turks and Caicos Islands for work. My husband stayed with him after that."

"Tell me about your experience with him while he was admitted."

"*My* experience?"

"Yes, what did you see in the management of his care?"

"My view of Jamaica while my son was admitted was that they had limited resources."

"Was the hospital equipped to care for his needs?"

"No, the hospital was not!" She became visibly upset. "There were a lot of children there, I don't know—they lacked equipment, space, nurses. They had to be reusing stuff."

"Was Raheim sharing a room?"

"He was never *in a room*, Delpha. He was *in a cubicle*. There was no form of isolation there."

"How many kids shared that cubicle?" I asked in astonishment. I knew that with leukemia the immune system is lowered, and the patient's airway should be protected by way of keeping him from others.

"Maybe around four of them were there. If one coughed, everyone coughed. There were never any forms of isolation. The door was open and was only closed in the afternoons."

"I know you said that they shared things. Tell me what was shared," I asked.

"For instance, the oxygen tubes and masks that they used were washed and reused between patients. This included the mask and even the spirometer."

I cringed. This is a volumetric exerciser used for breathing therapy.

"Apart from the fact that it was an open unit and everyone was together, those things I did not feel good about," said Alicia.

"What about the care provided by the doctor and nurses?"

"I think it could have been better. I don't think the doctors and nurses were very attentive. They were not children friendly, nurturing, or loving. They stuck Rasheim so many times. When he cried, they did not talk to him lovingly. I expected more from this children's hospital, and I wish they had been more caring. Sometimes when a patient called the nurses they would not even come."

As Alicia shared this unpleasant memory with me, I recalled nursing in Jamaica. We had to reuse even the urine cups after we tested the pa-tient's urine for infections, which would be horrific for most nurses else-where in the world to imagine. I prayed to God to give me a better job because working under those conditions stressed me out. I felt limited because I could not care for my patients the way that they should have been taken care of.

Today I am blessed to work in the healthcare system of the United States. It feels like I have been through it all, and I can tackle almost anything

Oh, how I yearn to have the financial abundance to run the healthcare system in Jamaica. It would be one that is efficient to the core. No long hours of waiting before they can see a physician. Supplies would be provided for individual and single use. Nurses would not be underpaid or overworked because of lack of staff. I dream of leaving America to help my fellow brothers and sisters back home. If only it were possible.

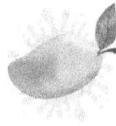

Power Thought

I have not worked in the Jamaican healthcare system for over ten years. The feedback from people who have visited often is that it was not good—in the sense that the waiting period is long, the hospital is full beyond capacity, there are next to no resources, the nurses looked tired, and it goes on. Working in Jamaica, I learned a lot.

Nurses in Jamaica are grossly underpaid. In 2010, I made approximately a net $1,000 per month in US dollars. ER nurses made more than the other nurses, who might make about $400 per month. By the time I came to the US in 2017 to work as a contract nurse, I brought home an estimated $2,400 per month. That was after they deducted money from my check to reimburse the international recruiting agency for the fees I was charged to be a part of the program. I was indebted to the organization for two years. I was not allowed to work anywhere else until that commitment was fulfilled. Even after the deductions, it was double my Jamaican salary but was meager by American standards.

We nurses, no matter where we come from, selflessly care about our life and death work. What I have witnessed while working in Jamaica is that we gave our best as nurses. We heard stories about the substandard care, and that was not my experience. I care deeply. Our hearts were present with the patients we served. Sometimes our selflessness goes beyond the call of duty, but that is the reason why we became nurses in the first place. It is the basis for our integrity.

Could the Jamaican government ever pay us for the selfless care we give? I would say no. They do not pay appropriate wages to nurses for what we give to our patients and their hospitals. Our integrity is priceless.

My experience working as a nurse in America is that we are sometimes understaffed. The hospital beds are full and the overflow of patients stay in the ER, or they are sent to the floor with a hallway bed with makeshift privacy while they wait for a room to come available. It is not easy working in most places as a nurse. There are simply too many sick people around to fit in the size of the hospitals being built. This has fueled my advocacy for preventative medicine.

Working in America comes with new challenges; however, will I allow these challenges to get in the way of me accomplishing my goals? No. I have a vision of where I want to go. I have a plan for how to get there, I have my *whys* and I stay focused. One reason is enough; I do not have to have a million reasons. Having even one reason allows me to remain committed.

Sometimes we need a *first push* from someone to get started, but if you have no one, learn to focus on your *why* and just do it. Five, four, three, two, one—move!

Part Three

Health Care: Misguided Cultural Mindset

Chapter 16

My New Life in the Turks and Caicos Islands

*I*left Jamaica in 2010 and traveled to the Turks and Caicos Islands for better wages and the chance to experience a different culture. Two new hospitals were being opened after they recruited a huge cadre of staff. The salary was twice the amount I received while working in Jamaica. The currency used was the United States dollar.

During nursing school, my instructor told us that we should give back a few years to working in our country before migrating. I gave back three years before I decided to move on. This decision to step out and leave home was not easy. I'd be leaving my strongly bonded family behind. Our connection to one another was just unbelievable; however, the birds must leave the nest to learn how to fly and so should I.

I felt a little guilty because the Jamaican government invested in me to obtain this nursing degree and I felt like I was turning my back on the system. Once I thought about it, the appeal of working in Jamaica on such a small salary would be a challenge for me to ever get ahead financially. Some Jamaicans did choose to stay despite the lower wages. I just needed something different, but it did not squelch the love I have for my country. If the country could offer higher wages, I might have been enticed to stay.

I packed my belongings and started my new life on Grand Turk in the Turks and Caicos Islands. This small island has a capacity for about five thousand people, so it is like a soap opera town. Everyone knows each other's business. The Turks and Caicos Islands are a British territory. This group of islands, also known as an archipelago, consists of forty different islands in the Atlantic Ocean south of the state of Florida in the USA. Only seven are inhabited.

On my first day on the island, we Jamaican recruits were so excited. A few of us came over from the same hospital in Jamaica and knew one another. We went to the beach as soon as we could, and I stood on the seashore and looked at how blue the seawater was. I could hear this swishing sound as the waves rushed against the rocks, and the sand was creamy clean; it squeaked when I took a step. I still could lie in it forever. I bent down and picked up a handful of sand and let it run through my fingers and smiled to myself—I knew I was going to love going to the beach. I loved going to the beach in Jamaica, but one was always far away, and this island gave easier access to the coastline.

We walked around, looking for a Kentucky Fried Chicken or some famous fast-food joint. We were informed that this did not exist. For fast food, we were told that we could go to the Poop Deck to buy fried chicken. I thought this was an odd name for a food establishment, but what the heck, we went with it. We were surprised to discover that the town consisted of some dilapidated old buildings. The government offices were in better upkeep. In the same proximity, you had a privately owned Mr. Cee's Supermarket that looked respectable. This was one of the best supermarkets on the island. It was clean and neatly stocked; however, it was crazy expensive. Structured beside this supermarket was the only pharmacy on the island. The other supermarkets were not well kept and if you are not careful, you might purchase expired goods. We were informed that fresh produce came once per week via boat from the Dominican Republic. There were a few more buildings scattered around, some for shopping for clothing. In the whole seven years I lived there, I purchased only two pieces of clothing. I was able to travel to Fort Lauderdale to purchase needed supplies. This was the case for many islanders. Clothing on the island was too expensive.

I found something rather interesting on the island while in the town one day. I noticed there were several ponds with a white frothy substance coming from them. When I investigated, the local people said they were salt ponds. These ponds were once salinas. The indigenous Taino people would gather salt and trade with the Hispaniola inhabitants in exchange for honey and fruits. In the late 1600s, they started exporting salt with the help of the British colonists in Bermuda. This salt was especially useful in the preservation of food.

One of my missions prior to working in the Turks and Caicos Islands was to complete my house that I had started to build in Jamaica. I worked and sent my income to Gina to supervise the completion of my house. Real estate is a big investment that I wanted to experience. I wanted to have something to go home to when I decided to leave the Turks and Caicos Islands. The Jamaican culture pushes you to return better than when you left. After leaving, if you are not able to return with or to something, to show that you were abroad, people will say that you went away and wasted time, even if those are the same people you were sending your hard-earned money back to. The thing is, people will often call you from home asking you for money to go to hospital or to buy food, and you will send it, but they will not remember sometimes that you helped them. You must return better than how you left, or you will be looked down upon.

The Turks and Caicos Islands provided a new world of experiences for me. My contract provided a three-bedroom house with indoor plumbing, a bathroom, and my own bed to sleep in. The mattress was sturdy and comfortable with no holes or insects. This concrete and cinder block structure felt secure.

In the one *cauya* bed of my youth, where I slept with two of my sisters, the mattress was made of springs cauya, made from the coconut tree husk, which was used to surround the springs to add comfort. After overuse, the springs stuck out and pricked our skin. We could do no better, for this is what poverty provided. Mama used old clothing to replace or stuff the middle of the mattress where it sank the most. Scorpions and bedbugs, called *chinks,* bred in the holes in the mattress and bit us from

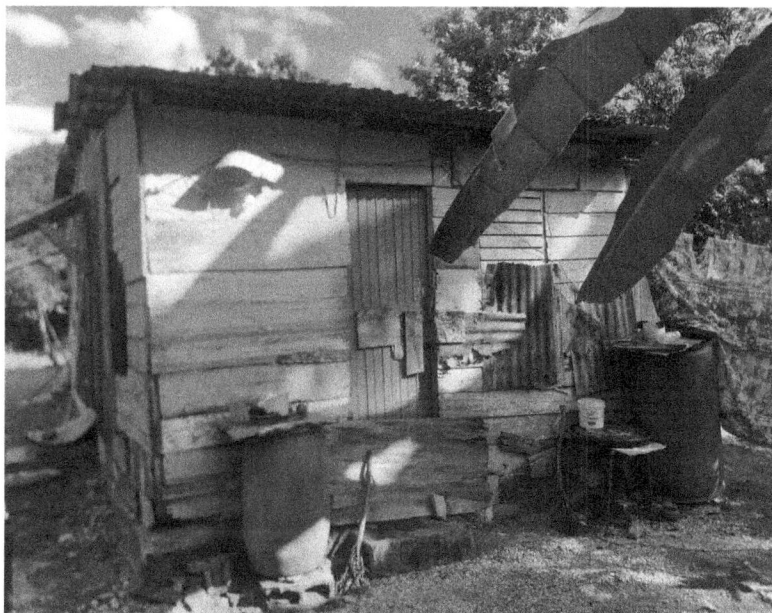

Image 14: Our home sheltered us from rain and provided a place to lay our heads.

time to time. The scorpion bites were painful, especially from the larger ones. Mama searched the bed at times before we went to sleep at night to make sure it was safe for us to sleep. It was just my life. I knew no different until I began to visit other homes in the church community and witnessed our differences with how we lived.

My sister Shelly often used my sister Donna's feet as her pillow to find comfort from her asthma. This helped us to fit on the bed. We usually lay close together, making it difficult to change position. It was a head-toe-head system until my sisters gradually left home and I had the bed to myself. Our roof was made of zinc. When the rain fell, our zinc roof leaked, so we had to put plastic over the bed with containers filled with pieces of old clothing to prevent splashes. Sometimes this was not enough because the rain still fell into the bucket and splashed over onto the bed. We could not afford to fix the roof. When I attended the university, I had to share a room with two of my girlfriends, Mitzie and Tanesha. We had a single and a double bed, and Mitzie and I slept on the double bed.

The boarded floor of our home was built over a cellar. The chickens and pigeons favored this cellar to roost and lay their eggs in private, away from their coops out in the yard. We kept all of our doors open except for the one to the backyard during the nice days, but when the rains came, and at night, we had to close the doors. The unbearable smell of the poop and urine scent filtered up to us, especially during the rains.

I took in a deep breath of fresh, Caribbean air. "Oh, there is no smell of pigeons or chickens here," I said to myself.

I looked at my new surroundings. This accommodation refreshed my soul. I had this three-bedroom house all to myself. I was amazed at the wonders of the Almighty, and I would not say that this was luck. I believed this house was an answer to my daily prayers, where I asked God for guidance and help.

We tend to forget about God when we are happy and only seek him when we are sad. In that time, we are not in need, but it's the best time to call on him because we can first thank him for those good times. It is at that time when we can ask him, with sincerity of heart, to continue to bless us in our joys. This house was a blessing and a joy.

"Oh, thank you, God, for my blessings," I said out loud as I toured my new place.

In contrast, the walls of my childhood home were made of board with peeling paint. Some areas were rotted down and had holes you could peep through. There was one concrete floor in the room at the entrance of the house, where we ate and where guests could visit. These concrete floors were cleaned and polished with a red dye and had a sheen that you could see yourself through.

The rooms that Papa added to the house later always had cement floors. We were barefoot and poor, but our bodies were never dirty or smelly. After taking our baths outside, we often used cut-open limes to rub citrus under our armpits for an additional layer of cleanliness. Those who needed extra lime were playfully referred to as green arm. It meant that you were extra smelly if you need more limes.

The Lord gave me the strength to reach this far, and he continued to bless me to reach even further than I could ever imagine. When I could read, I read everything in sight. These books helped to develop my imagination. How dare that little ghetto girl come and achieve this much—even to the point of becoming a writer. With God, our status does not matter. I cannot help but look back to see how far I have come.

These days I pray for wisdom, knowledge, and understanding. Nathan and I read the book of Proverbs together to learn these principles. In the great book—the Bible—Matthew 21:22 states, "Whatever you ask in prayer, you will receive, if you have faith." In this life we need only to call upon God and our cravings will be satisfied if we believe in him and it is his will for it to be done. The same is true for our worries. God is certainly bigger than those.

We had electricity, not because we could afford it but because, shamefully, we were able to steal from the light pole at the entrance to the lane. We used electrical cords that ran on the ground from the light pole to our home. We could not run these cords on poles because we'd be prosecuted if the police or the Jamaican Public Service saw it, as the

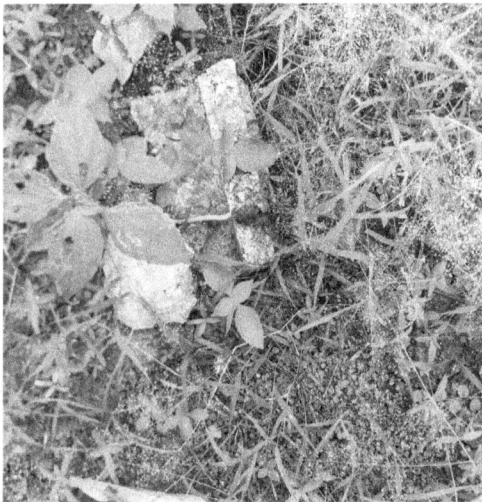

Image 15: Illegal electric wiring on the ground.

practice was against the law. We used black tape to cover exposed wires. This exposed area bubbled up and released steam through the mud. We made sure to jump over these areas when we walked by to avoid electrocution. We had no fridge or television at the time, and the light was often weak or dimmed a lot.

There is no justification for sin or breaking a law, and I am glad that God was gracious with us in our survival mode. As survivors, we did not always do the right thing, but I believe he knew our future and assisted us to the point where we were able to have the means to pay for electricity. Mama insisted that we do this. I can recall her concern and desire to do the right things in life. The Bible states that we should not steal, and this weighed heavily on her as a Christian. The burden of this was lifted when we were eventually able to pay for this service. It was so nice to see that we had electricity on a pole along the road just for us.

Every morning, we gathered lime, mint, lemongrass, cerasse, and soursop leaves for tea from the garden. God blessed us during those times. These leaves also kept us healthy with their medicinal benefits. I will always remember these days and thank God for guiding me this far. He is a powerful and amazing God.

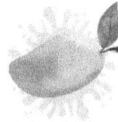

Power Thought

At times we are in certain situations that appear to be stressful, but God is watching over us. He knows our limitations and he wants us to gain strength from those trials we face. We all have something that may attempt to break us, but we must never give up and must continue to push through.

Take pride in who you are as a person. Do not succumb to your surroundings. Rise above them. I was reading Nathan his bedtime story one night. In this book, there was a little boy by the name of Jonah, but he liked to be called Joe because it made him seem older than his twelve years. He was at gym class and his coach said, "I need six pull-ups from all the boys." The boys all reluctantly started to do their pull-ups. Then it came to Joe's turn. He asked himself, *Will I be the weak link in the chain?* To make things worse, here came the class bully who always picked on him. This guy was huge. He did not even have to jump to reach the pull-up bars. He was able to do nine pull-ups. Joe began to really worry. Now the entire class had their eyes on him.

"Okay," he sighed with a deep breath, and he began. After doing one pull-up he realized it was not as hard as he'd thought. He wondered what everyone was so worried about. As he continued, the coach started yelling, "Unseen force!" Everyone got up and shouted, "Unseen force! Unseen force!" Joe was now at the tenth count. He continued … 11 … 12, 13, 14, 15, 16 … Joe started to feel the pain in his shoulders, but he did not give up … 18 … 19 … 20…. He could not believe he had done it. Simply awesome.

Joe did it!

Sometimes you have an unseen force within you that you need to harness to push you forward. People will try and distract you by putting you in a corner. The power is in you to step out. You may not have friends or family to push you or cheer you on, so be your own cheerleader. If somewhere down the line God sends someone to cheer you on, so be it. First develop that self-confidence. Do not allow your fears, or anyone, to keep you down.

Chapter 17

Meeting Nurse Jack

I do not remember the very first time I met Jack, but I can recall him asking me to walk over to the old hospital with him to collect some supplies. The hospitals were in a state of transition and needed supplies. We were all expected to stock the new hospital in preparation for the opening in a few weeks. This was an exciting time we all looked forward to—both the old staff members and the new recruits. We enjoyed getting to know one another in the process.

As I walked over with him to this new hospital, I did not have much to say to him.

"Please sit in the reclining chair there while I get the supplies."

That's strange, why would this guy ask me to join him to get supplies but ask me to sit in a chair while he gathered the supplies? I fell asleep while I waited.

"Wake up, Delpha."

Startled, I realized I had been there for a long while. "Sure," I said as I stood up.

As we walked back to the new hospital, he showed me the few things he had collected. "I found the forms we needed."

My eyes widened as I bit my tongue. I did not have to come with this man for some silly forms.

Everyone appeared to love him, well … almost. We will get to that later. He catered to the needs of the community, including the elderly and the Haitian population. We watched him work with patients and saw how loving and attentive he was to their needs. At first, I was not interested in him in a romantic way as he looked much older than me.

I was eventually drawn to his nurturing demeanor. He took good care of his patients and he moved with slow deliberation. All I saw when I looked at him was a guy with a protruding stomach. He moved with such an exaggerated slowness, it got on my nerves, and I really did not pay much attention to him. A coworker friend of mine who came over with me from Jamaica said, "Nurse Jack likes you, but you are not looking in his direction."

I found out later that my friend told Jack, "If you want to get her attention, just ignore her and she will come to you." He used that oldest trick in the book to get to me. I did exactly that; I drew closer to him when I thought he was ignoring me.

I began to admire his big, beautiful, brown eyes. When he looked at me, I felt I could drown myself in them. There was not a lot to do on the island, and I did not drive. He started to come over to my house and we'd go for walks, and I occasionally rode with him to shop for groceries. He quickly and freely loaned me his car when I needed a favor. He was from another Caribbean island, Saint Vincent, and the Grenadines. He had lived on Turks and Caicos twelve years prior to my arrival. To me, he was kind for doing so.

He talked about his past relationships, ex-wife, and his most recent past girlfriends. He seemed to undermine their character to make himself look good. He claimed that he divorced his ex-wife because she did not want to live in the Turks and Caicos Islands as it was too small. I found this to be an unbelievable statement, but I dismissed it. I had a nagging feeling that his stories did not add up. I knew that if I loved a man who treated me well, I would go with him anywhere. He did not seem to have gone out of his way to go visit her once he left. It later made me wonder how caring he really was.

He played the victim in these relationships, and my heart went out to him. I sympathetically fell in love with him. When I saw him, I lit up. He wooed me with promises to care for me. He made me feel like he'd give me everything I wanted. We made decisions together and were inseparable. I loved spending time with him, going to the beach or fishing.

At work, we ate our lunches together. I craved the attention he showered me with.

Jack eventually told me that he was going to marry me despite the reputation and rumors that preceded him. That was his proposal. He did not get down on one knee or anything. Of course, I wanted this as I was unmarried at thirty-four years old, but I turned a blind eye to his complete lack of romance. The church community that I grew up in stressed that you must get married by a certain age, that fornication is not acceptable, and all of my friends were already married. I wanted children in marriage with a man who cherished me. My list of rationalizations for the red flags around Jack was endless.

We continued to date for a year. For fun, we would go to the beach, plan events at each other's houses, or go to a restaurant. We made do with the lack of places available on our small island. I wondered why a man this age was not married or settled down. Over time, I discovered that he had a son with his ex-wife and two more children with two different women. He had a daughter with his last girlfriend who lived on the island and did not like him. He'd make comments like, "She looks like the devil." Several people commented that she was a "bad girl," so I believed him, but I also knew that there were two people in that relationship, so the fault had to lie with both of them.

Jack blamed all of his breakups on the other women. He usually said about his first daughter's mother, "All she was about was looking good." She was all about getting dressed up, desiring the latest hairstyle and cosmetics," he'd say, or, "My ex-wife did not want to come to the Turks and Caicos Islands with me because she listened to her mother, who advised her not to go as I am some wicked man, but she was also cheating on me," he said, or, "She was a woman that ran wild and was very worrisome," he'd say about the mother of his last daughter.

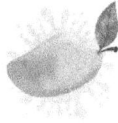

Power Thought

Love yourself first.

At this point, I did not think much of myself and did not know my worth. A symptom of that is when we accept negative behavior toward us. I eventually became aware that it was on me to take responsibility for my life and own my decisions as a result. But I was not learning from my mistakes fast enough because I learned as I went along. I knew enough that I did not want to repeat the mistakes. Or so I told myself.

Chapter 18

I Married Jack

We set a wedding date after living together for a year. I wanted to get my relationship with God in order. I did not want to marry Jack before he was baptized in the church. He grew up as a Seventh Day Adventist, so this religion was not new to him. He agreed to get baptized. Even though we lived in my apartment, we ceased sleeping together. I now believe he was patient with the process only because his sexual needs were met elsewhere.

"Jack, what about our rings?"

"I do not like to feel anything on my fingers."

"Well, Jack, I want a ring. How are we going to purchase this?"

"I have no money; remember, I have three kids to feed."

"You never have any money, but we can go to the Cruise Center and slowly pay down on my ring."

"Okay then, let's do that."

A friend of mine worked at the Cruise Center and with her help, we could get a good price for a wedding band. With my work at the hospital, I could not wear anything elaborate due to the risk of germs. The price of my 14 Karat gold ring was $634. Jack did not contribute the energy to help me choose it, nor did he contribute to the purchase. I was just too excited about getting married.

We traveled to the courthouse in Fort Lauderdale, Florida, for our marriage license. Of course, Jack had no money to contribute to our wedding ceremony either. He believed that if he had three children to take care of, I should pay for everything, including our wedding.

He bought an expensive camera two days before the wedding so that we would have nice pictures. The wedding ceremony was a small affair with twelve people. There was not one person there from his side of the family, not even a best man. His family, according to him, did not treat him well; therefore, he did not want to invite them. He often said that all they wanted from him was his money. The truth is, they were willing to come if Jack would pay for everything.

A Justice of the Peace performed the ceremony. Jack beamed as we said our vows to one another. I was elated because I'd finally married my baptized man, and things were right in the eyes of the church and in the eyes of God. I felt happy because finally, we could be that perfect couple. I believed that marriage would fix everything. My brother stepped in as Jack's best man and volunteered to pay for the reception at a local Chinese restaurant.

My wedding expenses were $2,000. This included my dress and poolside venue for the ceremony. I believed everything Jack said and falsely believed that marrying him would fix any doubts.

Out of his monthly salary of $2,800, $500 went to child support for his three children. He had credit card debt from buying things for other people. He claimed they did not pay him back and now he had to repay the debt. I never knew where his money went, but he wanted me to pay for all the other living expenses.

"Jack, you need to stop buying gifts for other friends—you are buying their friendship."

He was into the latest gadgets. Others often asked him to purchase things online for them as he knew where the good products were sold. Each time we traveled somewhere, he would give ten dollars to anyone who asked.

"Jack, will you give me ten dollars?"

"I don't have any money, Delpha."

"You never give me any money—what about our family? Do you feel the need to please people?"

He said nothing. There was never a response to that question.

After we were married, I told him he needed to contribute $250 every month for us to purchase groceries. He paid for this, but it was usually late. I did not see a problem with our roommate kind of living until I moved to the United States. My supervisor began to educate me more about a Christian money adviser named Dave Ramsey. Mr. Ramsey taught married couples about money management and how they should operate financially. My eyes began to open when I listened to him. I am ashamed to say that I overlooked every warning sign and quickly learned I was in this marriage all by myself. The pictures were not all that great either.

The first year of our marriage had happy times. We were communicating, going out together, fishing, saving—even though this stopped shortly after our wedding day. He had a credit card with a large interest rate. Instead of saving, I took part of the money to pay off his credit card. He did not like this and so he removed my name from his account.

We were trying to have a baby. Actually, it was more me than him. He was so shocked when I told him I was pregnant. I can remember the day that I did, I had to call him over the phone to tell him. On the island, word moves rapidly. I was at work one day and during the last part of my shift, I was going to see the obstetrician. He required that I do a pregnancy test. I really was not interested in doing so because I had already done one a few days prior. With skepticism, I did as he asked. When I saw one very bright line and the other one faint, I got so excited because I was finally pregnant after one year of trying. I could not contain myself. Others around me saw my smiles as if I were crazy. One of the nurses told me to call Jack to tell him before anyone else did. Remember, this is a town and island that is a soap opera. I called to share the news.

"Jack, I'm pregnant."

"Whaaat?"

I could hear the surprise in his voice. I convinced myself that he was happy with the news. At least, that's what I thought.

My pregnancy was full of back pains, and I still had to struggle to do all the household chores. I cannot ever remember getting a back rub from Jack, who was always out. He was a midwife, yet he did nothing to help me during this uncomfortable period. Some men often give their women back rubs. Not my husband. After having our son, he informed me that there would be no more children. It was not up for discussion. He would not have sex with me until I started using a contraceptive.

He was not close to his family because he thought they were dishonest and uncaring with each other. My husband grew up with his grandmother, whom he loved dearly. His mother would often visit him. He made contradictory remarks about my family. He often said that he liked how close we were and at the same time, he could not relate to our closeness due to his own experiences and would make negative comments about my family. I always wondered why he distanced himself from my family. Perhaps it was because he did not know how to be with a loving family, so he did not trust them because he could not trust his own family.

The relationship was not good. Throughout the eight years I was with him, we had several altercations. I remember packing my things to leave one Sabbath morning, but the church family got involved and I allowed myself to be talked into staying. We got so bad that one day we were fighting and our son, who was two years old at the time, witnessed my husband pushing me in the face. I packed up my things and flew to Jamaica with our son. If you know anything about Jamaica, you will know that working there was a challenge and workers are grossly underpaid. My sister Gina, who was building my house for me in Jamaica, convinced me to return to the Islands and to not allow anyone to take food out of my mouth. I listened, and I should never have gone back to Jack. Let me clarify this; she did not say I should return to *him* but that I should return to work there. Sometimes when you can get out, run and never look back.

At that time as well, we decided that we were going to take one of his other children's mother to court as she physically abused her in front of everyone at the hospital over an accident that occurred with another family member, His daughter was eleven at the time, and she came to live with us during the court proceedings. I took care of her, and she started coming to my church. She even got baptized, but she decided with the court to go back to her mother. This was disappointing as I started to really love this child. It was a challenge as her mother was not an easy cookie to work with, but I tried.

My husband often accused me of not attending to his other children, but I often asked myself the same question about him and asked him what else I needed to do. When he suggested that I ask how they were doing, I started doing so. He has a son and another daughter living on two different islands. Up to this day, I still don't know what else I could have done. One daughter I took in and cared for until the court decided that she had to go back home to her mother. The other one I brought to America and helped her to get a job so she could stand on her own. I did my part the best way I knew.

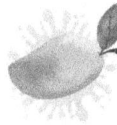

Power Thought

I have my perspective and Jack has his perspective about what went on in our relationship. Then there is what really went on.

Did Jack know how to be a father? Did I know how to be a stepmother to three kids who I did not know, two of them living thousands of miles away? I don't want to make the same mistakes again if I am given another chance.

The biological parent must take the initiative. Show interest in taking care of your children, then the stepparent can take a step and assist. Everything should not be left on one parent, be it the stepparent or biological parent.

This is what happens when we play God in our own lives. It's what happens when we pray a prayer and tell God how to answer the prayer. This is what happens when we fail to let God be the Lord of our lives. We make mistakes because we are competing with God because of our pride.

Chapter 19

Nurse Jack Falls Ill

I lay in bed waiting for Jack to come home from work at the hospital. My cellphone began to ring and vibrate in my hand.

"Hmmm, this better be Jack. Hello?"

"Hi, Delpha, it's Dr. Benjamin."

"I know your voice. What's up, Dr. Benji?" I loved working with her.

"I have Joseph as a patient in the ER, but it's nothing too serious."

"What happened?" I was more alert.

"His heart started to beat a little too fast and we are running a few tests, but you don't need to come—"

"—am on my way."

I hung up on her and dialed my girlfriend Brooksy.

"Brooksy, Jack is in the emergency room as a patient, and I need to go over there. Can you keep Nathan for me?"

"Oh God, what happened to him?"

"He is having palpitations. Can I drop Nathan off at your house?"

"You don't need to ask."

"I'm on my way."

What is Dr. B thinking? Am I not to come over? Is she crazy? I dressed faster than usual.

As I placed my six-month-old son Nathan in his car seat, he smiled as he stirred awake. I loved this little man's smiles. They always melted my heart. "Come on, little guy, let's get you buckled in here so I can go check on Dad."

I jumped into the front seat, started the engine, and sped over to Brooksy's house. I pulled in front of the fence, where Brooksy stood and waved.

"Oh, thank you for watching him," as I ran to her and handed Nathan over still buckled in his car seat.

I was grateful for Brooksy. We kept supplies for one another's children on hand as we babysat for one another to save expenses.

"Go, get out of here. Let me know what is going on."

As I headed toward the hospital, I recalled when Jack mentioned his heart racing a few days before, after he had to medevac a patient to Jamaica. As a nurse, he performed a carotid sinus massage—a type of vagal maneuver—on himself. This is done by applying pressure below the angle of the jaw in a circular motion to slow the pulse rate. Jack said that he had success by massaging one side. I advised him at the time to see a doctor, but he refused. I felt guilty that I did not press the issue further with him.

The short drive to the hospital was the longest five minutes of my life. As an ER nurse, I could not help but play scenarios in my head about what I might see when I arrived. I tend to look at the worst-case scenario first. Doc Benji said it was not serious, but I knew it could be supraventricular tachycardia (SVT) again, which is when the heart beats abnormally fast, greater than 150 beats per minute. The normal heartbeat should be between 60–100 beats per minute. Supraventricular tachycardia could be treated with vagal maneuvers, chemicals (medication), or electrical cardioversion to reset the heart's normal rhythm. I recalled patients describing this as being hit by a truck in the chest, but it usually works. I also thought of atrial fibrillation, which is an irregular heartbeat. If it's new, that is, it occurs within 24–48 hours, then the electrical cardioversion is an option. If it's longer than that, the patient could be treated with a betablocker medication to slow down the heart rate. Electrical cardioversion depends on if the patient is stable or unstable. The cardiologist makes this decision. The problem with this scenario was that we had no cardiologist on the island, and the heart, in a case like this, requires a rapid intervention.

My heart raced with so many simple and complex scenarios. I began to panic because I didn't know what we were dealing with. I hoped for the best. The causes of these cardiac arrhythmias could be stress, stimulants, or sepsis.

I parked the car at the emergency entrance and ran through the automatic sliding glass doors, heading to where the stable patients were normally seen. I saw out of the corner of my eye that the trauma room light was illuminated. I looked in that direction through the open door. My heart leaped because we left the door open after a patient was stabilized. Jack lay on the bed and saw me rush through the door. My tears were uncontrollable. His expression looked sad, and we both began to cry. I hugged him tightly. Nurse Brown was checking a reading on the cardiac monitor.

"I'm sorry, Jack, I am so sorry. I think I caused this because we were arguing a lot and I put you through too much stress."

He hugged me tight and cried in the crook of my neck.

Nurse Brown stood watching us sympathetically in our tender moment.

Jack was diagnosed with atrial fibrillation, stabilized, and transferred from our Turks and Caicos hospital to the Dominican Republic, where doctors performed electrical cardioversion to return his heart to its normal rhythm. He was sent home and placed on medications.

Some of these medications have side effects, such as lethargy and impotence. Jack asked if anything could be done about the side effects- , and the doctor added something safe to his treatment plan to see if that worked, but it did not. We tried romance later, but he trembled so much afterward, we were afraid it might harm him. I also thought he was too afraid to try, but he kept saying it was because of the medications. I took my marriage vows seriously when I vowed to love him in sickness and in health. I was committed to him in heart and soul until death did us part.

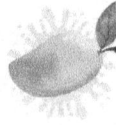

Power Thought

I was committed but he was not. Therefore, we could not function as a "we." Seeing Jack fall ill brought me to my knees. I looked at him in the bed and the question hit me.

Is this worth all of our fights? What is the purpose of living in this life if we are not loving and giving to each other? I don't want to continue on this path where we are always fighting.

When our loved ones are ill, sometimes this is when you get that either: You love them deeply and want to cherish what you have or you see old or new truths and need to break away to survive. Whatever your choice, do what will make both of you happy in the long term.

I *needed* to separate myself from the crazymaking.

Part Four

Freedom: Improving the Mindset

Chapter 20

Goodbye Turks and Caicos Islands

Before I began the application process, Jack agreed that we should leave together when it was time to live in America. His daughter Julia struggled to maintain a good relationship with her family and find a stable job. I wanted to help her to get to America, where jobs were plentiful. He mentioned once that he wished all of his children lived under one roof. This was my attempt to get many of them together. He did not object, but at the same time, he took no responsibility for the financial or emotional challenge of getting her to America. He wanted no stress at all. According to him, his doctor told him to avoid this stress as much as possible. I figured she was old enough to work and help herself after I got her settled. I also reasoned that as a Christian, I would have no problems with us living together. I filed the applications for all of us, including Julia, who lived in Saint Vincent and the Grenadines.

I did not file a case for his other daughter because an existing court order mandated that she live with her mother a few years prior. I also knew it was going to be hard to bring up a teenager with different principles and values from my own. I knew I would be left alone to manage the discipline because Jack always took the high road and left me to get the job done. "I will allow no one to stress me out. I will be dead gone, and they are still living and having fun," he said.

This was his favorite statement when one of his children's mothers called to complain about something his kids had done. I often encouraged him to spend time with his children in addition to the money he sent home to them. I never met his eldest son, who lived in Guadeloupe with his mother. Jack never introduced us over the phone the few times they spoke, nor did I ask. I did not know how to pursue that course and felt helpless. I believed that time with them was important, but I guess he wanted me to figure everything out while he agreed or disagreed with my decisions. It was if he expected me to be his secretary. I certainly was not his secretary.

I was tired of the arguments. I did not feel loved, nor was I treated with respect. He wanted to go, yet he wanted to ensure that I completed my three-year contract first in South Carolina before he could follow. He often said that our relationship would be better once we moved off the island as there were too many people trying to interfere with us. I tried to encourage him about the many jobs available that required minimal physical labor. He stood firm in his belief that his heart could not manage a job working in America. I also researched what advanced healthcare might be accessible in America compared to what we had on the island. I was concerned about the lack of medical resources on the island to give him the best treatment if he should have a cardiac emergency. He would have to be flown off the island for advanced care. In spite of the facts, he was not interested in relocation at the time.

Ultimately, Jack decided to stay in the Turks and Caicos Islands until I was settled in America with a stable job. I left him behind as I headed to America with our son, who was almost four years old. We agreed to put a pause on Julia's move with me because we agreed it would be too much for me to handle.

I took the State Board National Council Licensure Examination prior to my departure. Once I passed, the employment company ensured my skills were up to date and required a one-month training class before I could be placed. My family graciously supported my efforts and cared for Nathan during this time and ensured he made it to school and spent time with him.

As an international recruit, I was to live in the dorm and share a room with two other roommates while I prepared to commence work in America. This arrangement lasted one night. I did not like the living arrangements offered and chose to live with my sister, Miss Fearless (Marie) and her family in Ft. Lauderdale, Florida. She loaned me her car to drive to my training.

Nathan continued private schooling. During that time, my sister and her husband took care of us. Jack sent me five hundred dollars a month to pay for our son's tuition. I kept him in his private school because this was a familiar setting for him, and I knew I would move as soon as I was offered a contract.

Five months after my training, I was offered a three-year contract in South Carolina as a registered nurse. During our time there, I placed Nathan in public school. I quickly saw this was a mistake as he came home with scratches and bruises from bullies. I'd had enough when he told me he was hit in the face by another boy on the school bus. For the sake of my son, I vowed to let him remain in the familiar Seventh Day Adventist private school once we moved back to Florida.

I lived on a meager income after the company kept their percentage of my salary as repayment for immigration expenses. I attempted to understand the financial aspect of the American economy, in particular this thing called a credit score. I wanted to find out how to improve mine. I learned that the higher your score, the better the interest rates will be when in need of a loan. I fell for this because I did not know about any other way to accomplish my dream of home ownership.

I was informed that I should apply for and receive credit cards to build my score. In addition to the credit cards, I added a Wyndham timeshare to the balance. I justified the purchase with the thought that I was wise to leave it for Nathan. It was the worst financial decision of my life. The truth is, I was so desperate to break the cycle of the poverty I grew up with that I fell for these schemes and worldly advice. The Bible teaches in Proverbs 22:17 "The rich rule over the poor, and the borrower is slave to the lender." I was a slave to all of these lenders.

Yet, I did not stop there. A large part of that debt was the $18,000 loan I used to purchase a brand-new car. I really got into building that important credit score, my new idol. I even bought furniture on credit.

I have an ingrained phobia for debt and here I was with tons of debt. The Bible even advised me not to do it, so I should have known better. In the Jamaican banking system, I would never be permitted to acquire so much debt. They will not lend money or issue a credit card unless you have cash in the bank. I must admit, my preference is for this method. Here in America, it's different; one has no cash yet is given a credit card—several credit cards. My head ached and I knew I had to get out of this mess. I followed this worldly advice to the tune of $33,000.

Desperate, I searched YouTube for financial counseling and stumbled on Dave Ramsey, who I had listened to previously. His program caught my attention when he said things like going into debt for certain things was "stupid on steroids." I began to follow his Seven Baby Steps system and studied several of his books. I put what I learned into practice. I saved up my emergency fund of $1,000. Second, I began to clear my debt using his Debt Snowball. This is where I planned to pay off my debts from the smallest to the largest. Each time I cleared one debt, more funds became available to pay toward the others. In theory, this is supposed to quickly reduce the debt. I earned $26 an hour at the time. I worked extra overtime to make as much money as possible to put toward the snowball. It was easier because my mother already lived with me and cared for Nathan while I worked. My husband continued to contribute five hundred dollars when he could each month toward our son's expenses.

I saw rapid results. I was on my way to clearing my debts. My supervisor, Sandy, helped me to write down my expenses on paper. I realized that my expenses exceeded my monthly income by almost 300 dollars. We discussed what I might get rid of to balance my expenses with my income. I stopped Nathan's swim lessons and stopped going out as much. I found ways to save a few dollars from my food expenses. I was never big on shopping for clothing or things like that, but I faithfully worked my envelope system. This system kept me on a cash basis and I stopped using the credit cards. I labeled each envelope for what was in my budget: tithes, food, clothing, entertainment, and other anticipated expenses. Once an envelope was empty, the spending stopped. I recorded every dollar to the final penny. Peace and contentment replaced my worries and fears. It was a start.

My next step was to build three to six months of savings for expenses. After that, my goal was to save 20 percent of a down payment for a home with a fifteen-year mortgage. From there, I could save 15 percent of my income for retirement. Eventually, I would save for my child's higher education, pay off my home, build wealth, and give to others. This became my new plan. I quickly learned that if I owed money to a master, I could not build wealth. My hard-earned money would no longer contribute to the wealth of others due to any "stupid on steroids" behavior of mine. I have finally learned financial wisdom from some painful choices. It was on me to own my problem.

I was happy when my three-year contract was reduced to two years. The pay was meager, and it offered me freedom to look for work that paid a better wage for my credentials. When it was time to leave South Carolina, I owed only $7,000 on my car. At this point, I was almost debt free and a bonafide, debt-free-living evangelist.

During my tenure in South Carolina, Jack had a successful cardiac ablation for his arial fibrillation. I wanted to be by his side while he organized his surgery in the Cayman Islands, but he did not allow me to come because we did not have the money for the trip. According to him, the decision to do the surgery was sudden. I became suspicious because I thought a married couple should support each other. It did not sound right to me.

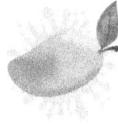

Power Thought

Jack did not want me at his side, especially at the time of his illness. That was a hurtful truth for me. I think we tend to need our loved ones the most when we are ill or have a realistic need to be met. My eyes were shut but my soul saw the red flag. Now, I'm making up for lost time. Don't ignore the red flags in any relationship, but don't focus too much on fear either. Whether it's an emotional or financial issue you're facing, try to attack it together through more communication.

It is important to set financial goals and follow through. It may start by simply putting yourself on a budget and ensuring you stay accountable to it. The envelope system sure kept me on my path. When I was finally out of debt, I spent a lot more on myself with contentment, knowing that all the needs were met first, and it allowed me to save a little more. As my income grows and I live below my means, I would like to get to a place where I can save over 50 percent of my monthly income. I think this is a wise savings plan because I have had a lot of setbacks while I've worked to get out of poverty. I learned about the Dave Ramsey system later in life, but we all have to start somewhere.

If I look back to what I have accomplished, I can see I have come a long way from that little girl Delpha who hated the feelings of hunger that came with the poverty she lived in. I have changed my mindset and continue to look forward as I work hard to make up for the time it took me to accomplish all of that. It just takes commitment, discipline, patience, and time to see the fruits of my labor. I need to remember to have fun along the way.

Dave Ramsey says that debt is the number one killer of the ability to save. I would like to add that this is true, except for when your income is much higher than the debt. When you owe no one, it is easier to save. It is also wise to note that it is not always the flashiest set of material things that we should aim to purchase as these are usually the most expensive. Live below your means. It's my mantra. Invest your savings in real estate, stock, or anywhere you can make an additional income. This is always the smart way to go. Side jobs, hobbies, or overtime are good places to start finding the extra money to put into savings. Do not use up your savings to purchase a liability. Use it to generate income and then you can splurge from the profit a little on some material things and not go broke doing it.

Chapter 21

Jack Finally Joins Us

When Jack finally decided to join us after we moved to Palm Bay, Florida, I encouraged him to save the money to pay for Julia's required medical expenses in Jamaica prior to their departure for America. I planned to pay for his daughter's travel expenses once the medical work was completed. The medical examination is required prior to entering the United States in the country of origin. In their case, it was Jamaica.

We set dates for them to meet in Jamaica a few months in advance. I traveled from South Carolina to meet them. As the day approached, I saved enough to purchase Julia's ticket. Jack was to cover his own travel expenses. Upon arrival in Jamaica, Jack informed me that he had no money. His story was that his employer did not give him his salary on time. It was so disappointing!

He had months to prepare for our plan. I desperately wanted us to work together. I had learned from Dave Ramsey how financial management should work in a marriage and this was not it. I was furious and felt betrayed because he did not live up to his part of our agreement.

His financial self-centeredness and lack of timely communication were apparent in this critical situation. I was done lending this man money without repayment. After all, Julia was his own daughter. Julia may not have known who her father really was, and I felt the betrayal on her behalf. I pushed back. I told him I had no money, and I was not going to use a credit card. I knew I would have spent the cash on him but with my new healthy way of thinking, I refused to consider using a credit card because I knew he would not pay me back.

We considered rescheduling the medical exam for when Jack had the necessary funds. I was not giving him a dollar, and I stood firm. We did not reschedule it because the cost of the overall trip would increase. Eventually, he borrowed it from my sister Suzan. I was disgusted over the fact that he had to borrow money because it made us look incapable. I knew I was capable because of my new knowledge but that he was not.

"We can't keep borrowing money, Jack. We need to save and budget for things."

It was apparent that he thought I was the one who should pay for everything like I always had, up until now. This time, I stood my ground. I really had no money. And I was confident and wiser because of Dave Ramsey's teachings about how married couples should manage their money.

He managed the repayment of the loan with my sister on his own as I wanted nothing to do with it. I knew that he did not like to look bad in the sight of others and I thought he might learn a lesson from this. Suzan is the same as the Mafia—she's someone you want to repay. When she is coming for you, everyone will know. When his paycheck arrived, he paid her back.

My two years in America were not easy, and I was living on a tight budget. I was able to help save for part of his daughter's medical bill. I felt as if I were this man's mother, except he treated me like a roommate. I had to be the one to initiate the plans, discussions, and everything as the head of the household. I wanted him to be responsible, to wake up and let us start to plan together instead of on my own. It should have been "we," but he did not want this, and I began to wake up and see the obvious. I kept asking myself why I did not realize this sooner. I began to see what my mother must have experienced with my father. I was that child who grew up in poverty, and Jack's behavior was going to keep us poor.

Sometimes it's your partner's mindset that is damaging while at other times it may be their lack of action or desire. It is also worth a self-evaluation, to make sure you have no habits or limiting beliefs. I was working on our financial health for both of us. I wanted our marriage to succeed!

What was Jack doing with all this money? I began to suspect that he might be funneling his money to other accounts in Saint Vincent and the Grenadines, plus the Turks and Caicos Islands. One cannot be earning as much as a nurse and be broke. It does not matter how many girls you have and are giving money to, or how many children you support, and I knew that he wasn't saving for the day when he would no longer be able to work. I could not figure this out and realized how different our thinking was. In fact, it wasn't similar at all. This should not have been a surprise to him because I shared with him what I learned in the Dave Ramsey classes along the way. He claimed he did not like that method and stonewalled the process.

Julia and I communicated often over the phone when she lived in Saint Vincent and the Grenadines. She informed me about her living arrangements with her aunt. She did not live with her mom because according to her, all her mother was interested in was men. I wired money to her for driving lessons. She spent the money on something else.

I informed her that she should try and save to help her in getting to America. She tried to, but her salary was not enough as she had to give the aunt more than half of her income for rent and could barely survive on what was left. I suggested that she discuss this with her aunt to see if her rent could be reduced, but her aunt refused to do so. She claimed her aunt was not a nice person and referred to her in a derogatory way.

She moved back to the country with her mother, where transportation was not available for work.

In the years I tracked Julia's immigration papers, I never spoke to her mother. I shared this concern with Julia. Being a mother, I would want to know who my child will live with. It was then that I spoke to her mother and her response was that she knew I was a good person based on what Julia had told her. I said okay then, and we exchanged numbers.

I first met Julia at the Norman Manley International Airport in Jamaica. I saw this very innocent-looking young lady knock on my car window.

"Hi," she said. She was dressed in an oversized orange blouse. I fell in love with those big, beautiful, brown eyes of hers instantly. She looked just like Jack. During this first meeting, she seemed to be very reserved. She came for her medical examination and then joined me later in South Carolina, toward the completion of my contract.

I have nieces and nephews who I love dearly, and no matter what they do, I cannot see myself associating derogatory terms with them. The saying is that if you want to know a true person, you need to live with them. I lived with Julia for six weeks, and things became very clear.

At the time, I lived in a two-bedroom apartment with Nathan and my mother. I bought my mattress from Amazon and another complete bedroom set from a local furniture store. I gave her the bed to sleep on while I slept on the mattress on the floor. We planned to move in the next couple of weeks to Palm Bay.

I told Julia she needed to find a job in South Carolina to take care of herself and that I was committed to helping her with the other things. I paid the rent and bought food. I taught her to do a budget, with an emphasis on avoiding borrowing money. I did not want her to make the same mistakes I had. I paid for her Permanent Resident Card, assisted with her social security number application, and took her around to look for a job.

She found a job, and I taught her how to drive. Julia did not show much interest in learning how to drive. I had to force her into driving lessons when we could fit them in until she was able to get her license.

I worked twelve-hour shifts and worked overtime to pay the extra expenses with one more mouth to feed. Prior to her arrival, I spoke to her father and asked about his contributions toward her. He once again said he had no money. When she arrived in South Carolina, I did not bother to ask him again, nor did he volunteer to help her. I was happy I had two of Jack's children under one roof.

I am not making myself out to be a martyr, but I grew up in an extremely poor community and I just wanted to do for others what I wished could have been done for me.

When you grow up poor, you are very aware of others who need assistance too. I would often try and find food out of a garden that my father planted to feed my brothers and sisters. I liked helping while growing up.

Julia arrived a few days before her twenty-first birthday. The day before her birthday, I quickly called her mother and asked what type of cake she liked. Chocolate, she told me. She told me that what I was doing for her daughter was so nice. When Julia arrived in South Carolina, she had a phone with a cracked screen. I decided to go to T-Mobile and purchase a new one for $200. My mother, son, and I excitedly sneaked into her room on her birthday morning to surprise her with these gifts. I felt a little deflated when I observed that she was not appreciative of the type of phone that I purchased. Honestly, I was very surprised.

She came to me one day and informed me that the phone was not working properly. We returned to the phone company and there they explained to us that she needed to purchase more data. This cost an additional thirteen dollars. One day while working in the ER, I received a text from her stating, "Please return the phone and take back my money because it is not working properly." The phone company told me nothing was wrong with the phone but that it needed an additional data plan. I confronted her about this, and timidly she admitted that she wanted an iPhone. I couldn't believe it! Here I am barely surviving, and this young lady's interest was solely in material gains.

I worked twelve hours a day in an emergency room, which was no easy task. I worked overtime for us to survive. She did not understand how we had to work together to meet expenses. This meant that we could not always have the perceived luxury items but needed to settle temporarily with the bare minimum to survive our transition to America.

I first entered the field of nursing because I wanted to help my father and quickly realized that it became my way of getting out of poverty. I had to make sacrifices and work hard, not just for a week or a year but every day, for many years. The cycle of poverty can be broken at any age if we make such sacrifices and learn as much as we can about how to manage money. Breaking means not just paying it off and doing it all over again but actually breaking it.

The knowledge I now possessed went against everything within me to purchase an iPhone for my stepdaughter. Yes, I possessed my iPhone before she joined me, which was purchased before I knew about smart management of my finances. I was stuck with it because I'd made the wiser choice to pay down the loan on my car and forgo the upgrades. All she saw was that I had an iPhone and felt entitled to have the same without a realization of the value of money. Guess what? It was now my job to teach her what I know about money management.

Julia implied that she wanted an iPhone but looking at her overall behavior, it was not in line with my own and I didn't feel as if it was good stewardship to do that. I exposed her to Dave Ramsey's teachings about smart money management. I needed her to be supportive of our goal so we could work together. I exposed her to the knowledge of how to make a budget. She now knows that she has a choice to live below her means so later she can have the life she wants without the weight of debt on her shoulders. This is a heavy burden that can be avoided because I know the pain of this very well.

I refused to buy her the phone. I wanted to teach her how to fish so that she could eat for life instead of giving her everything she wanted. I paid for her to start her nursing career through enrollment in the Certified Nursing Assistance (CNA) Program. This helped Julia to receive an income so she could grow financially. My hope was that she would achieve the highest degree of nursing possible in this field and be a registered nurse (RN). I could easily see that she was capable of attaining this and wanted to give her some hope so she could learn to dream, as I had. Today, Julia is self-sufficient.

Another reason I went into nursing was to ensure I could take care of myself. It does not end here. I save my money now. One can earn a million dollars for the year and still be poor. The choices I make now will lead me out of poverty, no matter what the level of my income may be. The fact that I have a nursing degree ensures my income.

It is up to me now to do my best with my new knowledge. My dream started with a move to America and to be free from the clutches of poverty. It is on me to own me. I am responsible for my choices.

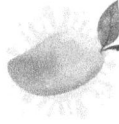

Power Thought

If you teach a man to fish, he will forever feed himself. Stop the enabling.

Not everyone will appreciate the sacrifices you make for them. After giving kindness, do not expect a reward. Maybe I expected one, especially in my marriage. Accept life for what it brings you at times and learn and grow from it. Would I have taken Julia to this country if I knew who she truly was? I know me and yes, I would. Sometimes I think I am too giving but am now learning to tailor this.

When you give, there is a peace within that you are contributing to the greater good. No matter how small it is, give. God blessed you. Why not bless someone else?

Chapter 22

Betrayal

Jack arrived in Fort Lauderdale, Florida, on September 2, 2019. He went there because at the time there was a Category 4 hurricane heading toward us in Palm Bay, Florida. He had to stay with my sister Marie in Fort Lauderdale, two hours south of Palm Bay. We decided that she would meet me halfway between the counties when he arrived. She knew the depth of my desire to see him. When he arrived, I hugged him so hard. I wanted to kiss him and rip his clothes off and do all the things boiling inside me. Instead, I was disappointed because this gentleman did not hug me as tight as I hugged him. He was not as excited to see me as I was to see him. Yet, I convinced myself that it was because others were around and he could not express his feelings.

When was I going to stop making excuses for someone who clearly did not love me? A friend told me that where men are concerned, I am naive, but this was way beyond naive. She wanted to put it in a nice way, but I have another name in my head that I called myself, and it was not naive.

We eventually moved in with one of my sisters and her husband in Palm Bay as he did not want to live in South Carolina. He did not like the idea of us living with family. He wanted us to pay rent, yet he only came to America with $2,000 in his pocket. Before he arrived, we discussed the cost of rent and what to expect. He was to save enough for us to do so. He initially did not come with Nathan and I to America due to limited cash flow, and we knew I would be on contract. He understood this. He left that responsibility to me, thinking that I would do this, as I usually did.

In life, we have givers and then we have takers. I wanted to stop giving without getting anything back. I wanted to stop feeling used. Jack was financially abusing me. I am now educated and stronger. I believe also that if I'd had knowledge of what relationships should look like, I would not have forced myself to marry him thinking it was a way to legalize sex and have children. Living a happy and completed life is much more than this.

I recall a time when he told me that out of all the women he dealt with, I was the only one so preoccupied with money. Looking back, it's a statement a narcissist would make in an attempt to make a partner stop whatever it is they're doing. When he made this statement to me over the phone, I sent him a text telling him that the other women did not love him as much as I did. I wanted us to grow old together, to live and be happy without worrying about money. I thought long term and he thought in the present. The cultural differences between us became very apparent.

Here I was with a fifty-plus-year-old man with a heart condition, no savings (that I am aware of-), and I now had all this new knowledge and wisdom. I started to panic. Working in the health industry puts things in perspective, and I knew that anything could happen in a flash. Life is here one moment and then the next moment we are gone. Retirement was going to take a lot to prepare for adequately, and we had none. I knew he had a pension from the Turks and Caicos Islands, but how were we to survive on that? It was simply not enough. This was another struggle we needed to address.

The cash that he brought only lasted two weeks. He liked to spend, especially on gadgets. I made sure he paid for his immigration card (green card) and his driver's license first, which totaled about $600. He spent the rest on other nonessentials. We opened a joint savings bank account at a local credit union. I still had my individual bank accounts. I did not encourage him to open another bank account because the focus was for us to save 20 percent, which would be $34,000 over the next ten months. I started the process before he came into the country.

We went to the builder together so he could see what was going to be built. With both of our incomes, a new home was achievable. Our expenses were low. We were not paying rent, only utilities and Nathan's tuition and food. He got his gratuity a few weeks prior to coming, which was at least $7,000. I discovered later that they gave him cash from the party they threw for him, but of course he never shared this information with me. What he did share was that he had to pay his daughter's college tuition and that was all that was left.

He made more money than I did, yet he said that he never had any money. My sister and husband gave us one year to live with them because the construction of the house would take only ten months. Thank God for family!

He eventually got a job with a visiting home health agency. I worked night duty at the time and requested to transfer to day duty. The nights were brutal. I could hardly hold myself up as I wanted to sleep. My husband's hours were 8 a.m. to 5 p.m. weekdays and he would be off on weekends. I would leave home at 6:15 p.m. and be home by 8 a.m. This was a problem where transportation was concerned with only one car.

We tried this for a week, but my husband would often be late for work, so we came up with a second plan. I suggested he drop me off at work and my sister could pick me up in the mornings as she worked close by, or I could take the bus home. He refused and began to behave badly because he did not want to live a life of humility nor live within his means.

He wanted us to buy a car using my little savings. This was a man who supposedly had no money. I suspect he just didn't want to be bound to a schedule or any kind of relational teamwork. Reluctantly, I took $3,500 out of my savings to buy a car. When we went to the car dealership, we decided that we were going to up that by $6,000 for a more reliable car. I am ashamed to say this, but I still had one more credit card which I used to pay the $1,500 down payment.

I do not believe in credit cards, but the lending company for the house informed us that I should not close this one. The following week after getting paid, I paid off the credit card. The company gave us the car with a thousand-dollar balance remaining, which was to be paid within a month, which we did when he started to contribute financially.

We started working on the budget together. A part of my salary would go to savings. After two weeks of working, while the family sat at the dinner table, Jack came home one evening with his belly full. He did not want any dinner as he had gone to a Jamaican restaurant and bought goat curry there. The dinner in front of him that we'd labored over, with him in mind, was pushed aside. This was a surprise to me because we had no money, and he had packed a lunch. I asked him where he got the money. He nicely informed me that a social worker he worked with loaned him $20. I was appalled by this. We argued because he didn't see it as a big deal. He was nonchalant about borrowing money from a stranger and I was disgusted by it. I was trying to live up to a certain standard and here this gentleman continued to borrow.

To make matters worse, they had a gift exchange at his work. According to him, he had no time to pick up a gift, so he asked the same social worker to purchase one for him and he would pay her back. I was suspicious. I should not have to say that when you are married, there should be a distance kept with other women. Jack did not have male friends. He was always around women, so that was another red flag.

The first two months after his arrival were good, not the best but good. They were good because we started to save and budget together, which was new for us. He started going out with Nathan and me instead of always saying no. It was not that great because there was still no sex or intimacy. I can remember him telling me that the feeling returned in Turks for a while, but it was now gone.

"And you did not tell me?" I would have jumped on a plane to see him. The sexless marriage continued, and I was getting frustrated. "Jack, what do you want me to do? I crave you! I am burning with desire."

"I am fine. Hold off on this and let us go to sex counseling."

I was not interested in sex counseling because I could feel something else was going on, and when a woman knows, she just knows. "What's going on with the social worker you work with? You visit her during the week and on weekends."

"We are just friends," he said.

"You brought a broken table home from her house."

"She threw it out, so I decided to take it."

I knew that this was a lie because about six weeks later, he came back and told me he was taking the table back because she got a bigger apartment. I did not respond, even though I observed.

I said nothing to him because I was tired of this behavior. He was no gentleman, and he was certainly not a devoted husband. I guess he thought if he could find someone to use, why not? I put it out of my mind and went to bed, and that night I had a very vivid dream. I dreamt that he was sleeping with someone. I believed God was sending me a message, yet still I played dumb after I woke up. I said nothing to him because I knew he would deny it, as he denied everything. I went to kiss him with our usual peck on the lips when he came home later that week. He moved away from me so fast, claiming that his mouth was dirty. It was such a strange response. Was that a smirk of contentment on his face I saw there? God spoke to me and all I could hear was the voice saying, *He is sleeping with someone.*

One morning he said to me in an accusing tone, "Your phone pinged all night."

Is he trying to say that I am seeing someone else? I picked up the phone and showed it to him. "Shelly is the one who was texting me."

Silence. It all became so clear then that he was using tactics to create conflict, perhaps to feel better about his betrayal.

He was looking for war and something to blame me for so he could walk out on me. He did not have the guts to say that he was done.

In retrospect, I sometimes wonder why I was so desperate for him to come to America. We had a different setting but the same old games. There were better men out there who would cherish me, but I refused to indulge in sin. Believing in him was stupid on my part. The signs were all there. God showed me the obvious and I chose to ignore it. I must therefore suffer the consequences of my naivety, my failure to see what everyone saw except for me. The depth of my stupidity was worse than naive.

Sometimes I think he hated me. I remember painting my house in Jamaica. The look of disgust when he saw I had paint all over me was obvious. He did not say, "Honey, let me help you take the paint off your face and hands," like a loving husband would do.

The next guy I marry, I want him to be able to see through my soul and care about everything I do because he will understand why. The Bible speaks about being unequally yoked. This can happen on so many different levels. Our value system on money was different; he believed in borrowing and I did not. I believed we should save together; he wanted to hide and save by himself. He carried over the behavior his whole life. According to Jack, his wife used up all his money and did what she wanted to do with it. He no longer trusted in family or marriage.

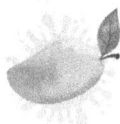

Power Thought

Marriage is about trust, commitment, and love. There was none for me. We were not on the same page in the things that mattered. It became painfully obvious that I was the only one interested in this relationship. Why stay with someone who does not want you around? At first, I rationalized things. "Yeah, it's just in my head but no…" How long can you fool yourself? It took me four months to finally let go. Jack deflected or found fault with me and instigated an argument so he could find reason to leave the house. If you find yourself in a no-win emotional situation like this, it's bound to hurt. You will often feel frustrated and long for answers.

Have the courage to choose you. Know when you can give no more, and don't expect to have the truth revealed. No one will value you like you can. If there is a man in your life who treats you with all the love he can, return that love and give him the respect he deserves.

God spoke and I heard his voice, yet I did not have the faith at the time to believe in him, to obey his Word. Now I suffer the heartache that goes with the consequences when I did not listen and chose to ignore the red flags. Jack did not value our marriage; he did not value me as a person.

Dreams, hopes, and wishes are all useless in a situation such as this because they change nothing. When a man feels like there is better out there, maybe there is better out there. After all, I know I am far from perfect. All you can do is wish them well and let them go.

Do not burden yourself or think that you are not good enough like I did. It is a waste of time. This will only tear you down, break you inside, and leave you thinking less about yourself. This is a toxic way of living.

Love yourself enough to run from situations like this. Especially don't marry into one like I did. Value no man above yourself. Put God first.

Chapter 23

The Meeting

Our marriage never had a good foundation to stand on. The deceit, the lies, were all there before we got married and continued. Our priorities were different, more so now than ever because I had grown stronger. The things I once accepted out of ignorance, I no longer allowed.

Jack began to bring home a lot of paperwork. Initially, he worked in our bedroom for several hours. Eventually, he started going to a local Barnes and Noble bookstore; at least, that is what he said. Sometimes he would say he was going to his colleague's house, and once he took our son with him. I discovered later that the "colleague" was the same social worker he'd borrowed money from before. When he was at home working, he often had to complete the paperwork for up to five patients, which took one hour each to complete. He consistently pointed out to me the time it took to complete the work. He was absent from home all day, returning later and claiming he'd only completed two or three of his files. I could not help but be suspicious of his behavior because things did not add up.

Maybe he did not care what I thought, knowing that it frustrated me. Did he want me to be frustrated to the point when I asked him for a divorce? I later discovered that this was his style when he wanted out of a relationship. He would frustrate you because he did not want to be the one to have to say what he wanted. Historically, he did not feel that he would have to pay for the divorce if he did not ask for it. I don't know why he did not cherish me or our marriage, and for a long time that bothered me . . . until I finally decided I deserved much more.

I did not like the direction our relationship was headed in, and I wanted to set things straight.

"Jack, we need to talk."

"Not right now—have no time."

"Then when?"

"Another time, Delpha."

It was always later with him. One payday, I checked our account to plan the budget, but his salary did not show in the account register, so I called him.

"Jack, I just noticed that your paycheck did not show in our bank account."

"That is what yuh called mi fah?" he said angrily and hung up on me.

When he came home that evening, I asked him the same question again.

"Is that the first thing that you greet mi wid?"

True, it was the only thing on my mind because this was the worst of my fears coming true.

"What happened to your check, Jack?"

"I stopped it."

"Why, Jack?"

"I don't want to talk about it now."

"Then when?"

"Not now."

This is a process called stonewalling. When someone doesn't want to answer you, they simply don't.

He walked out of the room. I brought the topic up again later.

"Jack, when are we going to solve this issue with your lack of contribution to our finances?"

"What are you talking about? I will contribute. Give me some time to work this out."

"I thought we were working as a team, Jack."

"Yes, we are, but I have no time to discuss this with you."

This hurt me deeply. I desperately wanted out of poverty and he did not care.

He made no attempt to comfort or reassure me. I could no longer fight for this one-sided relationship. It was painfully obvious that I was the only one who cared about our future together. This realization began to set in.

After two very long weeks, we sat down to talk. I thought I saw him trembling as he entered the room. I know I was angry and wanted to get to the bottom of this conflict. My list was ready.

"Jack, I don't like what has been happening. We need to sort these things out."

"You have a list; let's go over it because I do not have all day. Delpha, I don't have much life left. I want to live and enjoy myself."

"Jack, that is not what we agreed on before you came to America."

"I want us to be happy. Go out and have fun together as a family."

"This is what I want to talk about, Jack. You went behind my back and took your name from the account. Are you seeing someone else? Will you do marriage counseling? Will you be here for family time/us time? What about the name on the house? I added this because you were complaining and suggested I was keeping this from you." As far as I saw things, he seemed fine with whatever went on. I passed the list to him. "Why did you stop the account, Jack?" I waited.

"I stopped it for three reasons. I went to the bank to cash a check and I wanted to do a transaction afterward, and they would not allow it because I am not the primary account holder. Yet when we opened the account together, they told us that we equally have the same power over the account.

"Another point, I want to build credit. People have been telling me that I need credit, and for me to do so, I need my own account, so I can take out a credit card and you did not tell me this.

"And the third reason is that you called me and said that I could not get into the account myself—you told me that the bank teller told us we were both locked out. However, I was able to get in, despite this."

I could not help but roll my eyes at his answer.

"Jack, all a credit score does for you is put you in debt. But you were not interested in what I had to say because you claimed that you did not like Dave Ramsey, or that you do not have the time to talk. You could have said you wanted your own account, Jack. We could have done so if you felt so strongly about a bank account of your own. You did not need to go behind my back and do this. Furthermore, we agreed that the focus was to purchase a house so we could live on our own."

No faith in family, no faith in me. He trusted friends he'd known for four months over his wife of eight years. I have a good credit score not because I wanted it but because I tried to get out of debt by using the baby steps. When we needed to do anything, such as finalize our house purchase, my credit score could be used for this without him being stressed.

"I only owe a few thousand on a car loan, which I am working on getting rid of before we buy this house, Jack. This is *our* credit score, and we can use this to our benefit."

Was he discussing our private business and in the process putting me down? Did he not say to himself, "This is my wife, we are in this together, and she wants the best for us?" I'm sure now that he did not say this.

"I will continue to save toward the house," said Jack.

There was so much left unsaid because he never contributed a dollar toward our house savings.

"Jack, are you seeing someone else?"

"Delpha, I am not able to satisfy you. Why would I be with someone else?" He would not look me directly in the eyes. He used this sexual inability as a ruse, thinking I would not notice the obvious or question his motives. I recalled a time when I walked quietly behind him as he texted on his phone. When he realized I was behind him, the typing stopped and he put the phone down as he looked over his shoulder. I knew something was going on; I just didn't have proof.

He tried changing the subject.

"You are obviously not interested in my children because you don't ask about them."

"That's interesting. One son works and isn't speaking to you. Why?"

"Don't want to talk about it, "he said." Tell you another time."

"I helped one of your daughters who was physically abused by her mother," I countered. " You know I tried to help, but the court sent her back to her mother. What else could we do? What about your eldest daughter? I got her to America without any help from her or you. What more do you want me to do?" I asked.

"You did not invite Julia to Thanksgiving dinner two months ago." He was reaching for anything he could to demean me and make me feel bad.

"Jack, she had to work that day."

"You should have still invited her."

Jack realized I was too strong for him, so he could no longer push me into a corner. Plus, I have a host of close sisters to support me. He often complained about my sisters because I discussed things with them, and the result might be something opposite of what he might say. There might be some truth to this, and I justified it in my mind because Jack was not one I could trust my heart with. He did not like how close we sisters were. Plus, he didn't want anyone to know about his lack of integrity. Yes, the Bible says to leave your mother and father and cleave unto your spouse. I tried to do that, but things were not right. If I'd kept all this bad treatment to myself, I am sure I would have lost my mind. I needed the love and support of my sisters.

"Let's go to counseling," I suggested.

"I only want sex counseling," said Jack.

So, he didn't want marriage counseling, only sex counseling. He claimed we couldn't do anything in the house because it was not our house. He pretended to be so self-righteous, yet we had an entire half of the house to ourselves. I could not believe his answer. At first I thought he was ashamed because he could not function, but then I knew something else was up because he started to tuck the sheet under himself so that I wouldn't even touch him when we slept at night. Despite his lack of intimacy, I put his needs before my own. I felt that I would hurt him if I pressured him for sex because of his heart medication causing impotence. At this point, I only wanted marriage counseling because I could not imagine sex with someone who treated me like this, who I did not trust with my heart. I suspected he wanted to perform for a new girlfriend. He slowly isolated himself from me and our son and refused to spend time with us. He used that time to spend with his new girlfriend. Every time I suggested we spend time together, he claimed there was no place to go. One day we were driving in the car, and I said to him, "Jack, since you came here, we have been nowhere together as a couple. Look over there." I pointed to a restaurant-bar type of setting.

"That's nowhere to go, Delpha." That was the end of that discussion.

"I do not like the fact that we are building a house and I know nothing about the details of it. My name is not even on the title."

At every turn he had a different response.

"Jack, I explained to you that the real estate agent said that your name could be on it at the end when everything is finalized. Furthermore, when I met with the builders, you were at work."

He knew I was honest, yet he questioned my motives and integrity.

"Why did you not meet when I am off?"

"You did not give the impression like you cared to meet with the builders and myself. Furthermore, you told me that you had just started a new job, and you would not be able to take the time off. What more do you want me to do?"

This he said nothing to, and our meeting came to an end because he had other things to do. A week later I asked him for $2,000 to put toward the house savings.

"I don't have that."

"What do you mean by this? " I demanded. I was truly shocked. "Then how much can you contribute?"

"I don't know. I will let you know."

He had been spending money we should have been saving from his salary. My salary would pay the bills and I would put his in savings. The remainder after the bills were paid would also go into savings. He wanted to give me what he pleased after he spent or saved whatever he wanted for himself, without me knowing.

This was the final straw. I told him I wanted a divorce, and this time I meant it. No more.

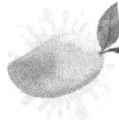

Power Thought

Jack did not fool me. I allowed myself to be fooled. I was dumb but now have seen the light. He wanted his name on my title for my house that he refused to contribute a dollar to. Why could I not see this at the time? Was I willing to accept everything this guy was dishing out at me? I thought I was not worthy to be loved, so I accepted all of this bullshit. I was so mad at myself. *Breatheeeeee.*

Everyone deserves to be loved and cherished by their partner. I am now dating, and I will not be with someone who will not give me what I need. This need I have inside is not about material things; I can do that myself. The things I need will be in his touch, will be in the beautiful things that a man does for a woman when he loves her. When there is real love, it can be felt. A woman knows when a man loves her and when he is playing a game. See it for what it is. Be open to who your partner is, and if this is not what you want and you know you deserve more, go. When you find the one who will cherish you, hold him tight and give him all that you have.

Chapter 24

I Divorced Jack

You wanted a divorce. Where are the papers? Give them to me and I will sign them," Jack shouted at me.

"That is not how it works, and you should know this. After all, it's not your first rodeo, Jack."

I had asked Jack for a divorce twice before and he would guilt-trip me. "Because you got your child, you want me no more, Delpha." Or, he would say, "Yes, I am no longer of use to you, so you do not want me." He never tried to change or improve his behavior because he needed to acknowledge that he was doing something wrong. In his mind, how could he be wrong when he was always right and had all the answers? He had four children with four different women, countless girlfriends, and many one-night stands. How could he possibly be right about everything? His behavior was crazy-making.

Another time, a text message appeared:

> EMAIL ME THE MARITAL SEPARATION AGREEMENT, YOUR FINANCIAL AFFIDAVIT, AND THE PARENTING PLAN SO THAT I CAN REVIEW THEM.

Ah, suddenly he is knowledgeable of what to do for a divorce. I wanted and needed a father for Nathan who treated his mother like a queen, with respect, as if I was the most important person in the world. I wanted Nathan to grow into a man who knew how treat his woman like that. I knew I had to make a stand for the sake of my heart and my son and leave Jack. My own father did not treat my mother like a queen. My sister Gina was especially angry with my father and spoke many times to the "other women" and told them to leave her father alone. Jamaican society, on the whole, seemed to believe that the women threw themselves at the men, whereas the men were the ones who allowed it to happen. And as such, I knew no better and was willing to accept this kind of treatment from my own husband for eight years. Now, I know what my mother probably felt like. I felt hurt, betrayed, angry, and broken.

There are many divorces because people fail to bother to compromise, to deny the self to comfort the other. Here I was with the same type of divorce. I felt as if I had done all the compromising in the relationship. He expected me to stay with him despite this kind of treatment. What was I to him? He wanted me to believe that he would be the breadwinner when, as the truth was revealed, it was his big lie. It was always a battle to get him to contribute to our household bills and supposed dreams. He treated me as if I stayed at home, was uneducated, and did not have a brain. To him, I was beneath him. If you're ever in a relationship like this, you may find yourself compromising to try to make the other person happy. But when you do that, you give up a little part of yourself.

My low self-esteem allowed him to walk all over me. As I became emotionally stronger and learned more wisdom, I no longer wanted to tolerate this behavior. He knew that I had low self-esteem. He cunningly worked throughout the eight years of our marriage to manipulate me and ensure my low self-esteem remained just that—low.

Finally, he really went all out on our way home from church with our son in the car. Jack shouted at me with rage.

"Jack! Remember, our son is in the car!"

"You started it, Delpha."

It was always tit for tat with him, absent of forgiveness. His attitude was, "If you hurt me, I will hurt you more." It always left me wondering what someone did to him that made him so calculated, cold, deceitful, uncaring, and unforgiving.

I started to see a counselor because I could not understand his behavior. He treated me like I was wrong all the time and told people I bossed him around to justify his displeasure with me, as if I could handle such a beast. He acted so innocent around others. When I asked him for a divorce, he often came home laughing and seemed happy. He seemed free, as if he was trying to make me see how carefree and happy he actually was now and that he was glad to leave our marriage, but he wouldn't leave. I actually had to ask him when he planned to pack his bags.

"Jack, when are you leaving?"

He immediately started to pack. "What about the money we were saving, Delpha?""

"I planned on giving you half of it, but now, I will not. I paid almost all of the $6,000 from my savings for that car you are driving."

He raised his arm in the air as if he were about to say something, then contorted his face. "Okay!"

Sometimes I felt as if he might hit me again, but I guess he didn't this time because other family members were around. Judith often said afterward, "I am glad you did not move into that house with him because the way how he looks at and treats you, who really knows what he is capable of?"

"Please, Jack, let's at least tell Nathan together and let him know that we are getting a divorce."

Silence.

"Can you at least wait until he leaves for school to start packing?"

"No."

I left for work that day only to discover that he told our son on his own that I threw him out of the house. The following day, Nathan was terribly upset with me. "Daddy was crying, Mommy. Why did you let him go? He told the teacher that you are no longer together."

I was sick of this man's manipulations. Did he not care about his son? I sat with Nathan and explained things as gently as I could. "Nathan, remember that Daddy and I talked about how we were not going to be married anymore because we were always arguing?"

"Yes, Mommy."

"You know, now we don't have to argue anymore because we won't be together. However, Mommy will not stop you from seeing your daddy."

I discovered how much I didn't know about Jack when we were no longer together. I've heard from others that the wife is always the last to know anything. I found this to be true when others started to come forward and admit they had been with him, witnessed something, or knew someone who was with him. He had not been faithful and the betrayal was worse than I ever knew.

This is partially my fault though. I knew about his infidelity, but I did not listen. I allowed myself to be influenced by his deceptive words because I wanted so badly for things to be different, or perhaps I was in denial. I held back because I feared things ending versus wanting the relationship to end because we would have to admit that we were not the perfect nuclear family.

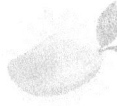

Jack was very vindictive; he knew how to hold a grudge and still smile with you. Two days after he moved out, he put a picture of himself lying in bed with a dog on him. He had moved into the social worker house, the one who he had said was just a friend.

One day someone told me that they saw Jack and a girl by the name of Miss Zelda kissing. I was not surprised. Of course, he lied about it after I confronted him, which meant that either he or our mutual friend, someone we both trusted and confided in, was lying. Which one was it? I already knew, deep down. Jack was willing to hold on to his lie at the expense of anyone else, even if it meant going against a loved one.

I hated how Jack lied about everything and how the friends and family around us including our child, slowly became aware.

I'd allowed this man to use me. Perhaps I should have been angry with myself, but I wanted to take my anger out on Jack for destroying our future together. I was angry and I wanted to get back at Jack, not just for this but for everything. But I decided to release that because the Bible says that vengeance is the Lord's, *not mine*. I wanted to heal from the effects of my anger, and I wanted to move past this experience in victory—with a new belief in myself and the ability to be joyful in the moment. Nathan was not able to understand everything yet, and I wanted to keep him safe.

After Jack moved out, I began my journey of discovery in counseling to figure out why all of this had happened. I wanted to know why Jack had treated me the way he did and acted as if I was the one who broke up our marriage because I felt compelled to ask for a divorce first.

First, I turned to the source of my pain to get answers, but Jack continued to shut me out. He viewed any contact with him as an attempt to get back together. My family could not understand why I still cried over him and texted this guy. I learned that my tears were not for him but for all the things I'd sacrificed in this farce of a marriage, and this was my consequence. I did not want him back; I only needed answers. Apparently, I was looking in the wrong direction.

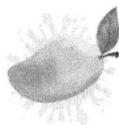

Power Thought

The truth is, I may never know the real reason why my husband behaved the way he did. I can assume that he fell out of love with me, but why not just walk out the door without all the drama? Why spread lies about me to others? But then again, he acted like a narcissist, so what else could be expected? I do not want to think about it anymore.

When I told Mama that Jack and I were getting a divorce, she started to tell me all of the things I had done for him and for his daughter to get to America, and that I should not leave him.

"Delpha, I can't understand why he is not grateful for all the sacrifices you made."

"Mama, they got what they wanted." I could tell she was hurting for me. "Mama, it makes no sense to stay in a marriage where I am not loved. It's not like your days when you had no choice with Papa. I have a choice and I'm making it. Dry your tears and be happy for me. I have a job, make my own money, and have an education that can't be taken away from me. I know how to take care of myself and Nathan."

Sometimes you have to use the mind God gave you in order to be your own hero. You must make the change you want to see in your life.

Mama finally realized that I was an independent woman, one she was unable to be like when she was my age. Our ways of living are completely different, and she sees how I have broken free from the bondages of our misguided cultural mindset. I had mixed feelings where I felt the joy of freedom, yet the effects of my mistake still stung. I knew it would just take time for my heart to heal.

Now I smile each day, having a sense of freedom, because I am now investing in the stock market and preparing for retirement. I can do me; I can budget the way I want to; I can plan for vacations; I no longer need to walk behind anyone saying, "We need to talk." I no longer have to hear, "Not now," and then the time to talk never happens.

I want to someday know the feeling where someone treats me as if I am the most important person in their life. We make time for those we are interested in.

Chapter 25

Answers to the "Why"

I needed to see a counselor to help me unravel this confusing relationship. It just blew me away that I could not have made my marriage work. I could not understand why this "gentle" man was so mean and unforgiving to me when he was the one who was cheating even before we got married. What did I do wrong for him to even think that I need forgiveness? He treated me like trash. How dare I tell him to move out when I was beneath him. In his mind, I should sit and take it.

I explained the ins and outs of our marriage to my counselor. I needed confirmation that I was not going crazy. I needed these answers because I wanted closure. I wanted to understand why I was so angry, and I wanted this anger toward myself and Jack to be gone. A page in my life had been turned.

After explaining everything to her, she looked at me and said, "Delpha, your husband is a narcissist."

"So *that* is what that is," I said. *Wow*, there it was—the answer to all my questions.

I began to research the topic. According to the Mayo Clinic, narcissism is a personality disorder in which the person is caught up in themselves and lacks empathy toward someone else, especially if they are not praised, despite all the good the person has done. This mental disorder could be linked to genetics or the environment, or it could be neurologic.

Of course, this was not an official diagnosis but feedback to help me understand what I might be dealing with. I couldn't have cared less about a diagnosis; I just needed to know I was sane and that I was not imagining things. I had an idea of his abandonment issues, and I do believe they stemmed from his mother, who saw him on rare occasions when she would look for him at his grandmother's home. Jack loved to be praised. He loved when I purchased gifts for him, but he never found the need to return the favor. He wanted people to see him as the perfect being, so he studied his people of interest and their supply, so he could start out by fulfilling their needs. When this was done, he had created someone who would worship at his altar. I stopped praising this man after all of his bad treatment. Throughout the years, I stopped jumping when he said to jump.

Suddenly, everything became crystal clear. I no longer need to text him and ask him why. He used this to say I wanted him back. Yeah, right. This is a characteristic of the narcissistic person who wants all the attention. He needed his ego to be constantly stroked. My counselor had vast experience in this field of narcissistic abuse and recommended resources for me to research further.

The answer to the question to why Jack would not leave is because the narcissists will feel like a failure if they leave. I asked him to leave because I could no longer endure the abuse and the abandonment in my marriage. I was faithful to this man for the entire eight years of marriage and it was not reciprocated or appreciated.

Have you ever been in the same situation? Read a book on passive-aggressive narcissists to identify them and to determine if this is a situation you're dealing with. It is my hope that you never experience one!

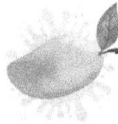

Power Thought

According to my research, Jack fits the description of what my therapist told me he was, a narcissist. I am not a doctor, and Jack has not revealed to me that he's had a diagnosis of being a narcissist. I am speaking to my experience only and to the resemblance of his behavior to the symptoms

I discovered in my research. I know why I felt so manipulated. It's be-cause I was manipulated from the time we met.

My brother-in-law told me that Jack did not have the approach to speak to a woman straight. He told stories to uplift himself and put his past women down. By doing so, he gained sympathy from his current interest and caused division between the ex and the newcomer, who was oblivious of his true nature and only saw his charms. He targeted women who were in a vulnerable position or had low self-esteem, and could easily manipulate.

He went to love bombing, where he would promise the person of current interest anything that she desired. If it was attention, he gave it; if it was sex, he gave it. Whatever she lacked, he became her knight in shining armor. He did not have a mind or personality of his own, he adopted the current woman's idea by wanting the same thing. He took on her needs and interests. The person he is interested in is usually calm and cooporative. I was like that at one point. I was compliant and easy to manipulate. Jack saw this—out of all the girls who moved to the Turks and Caicos Islands, he zoomed in on me.

I stood my ground whenever he hid his money. He developed a hate for me beyond my comprehension because he then saw me as someone who would no longer fulfill his needs. In an article written by Melania Tonia Evans, she points out that people with this type of personality dis-order love when you feed their egos. I chose to no longer feed Jack's ego. He put me down to his colleagues to receive sympathy. No one would believe that such a caring, soft-spoken, docile man could possibly be a manipulator.

I was drained. I could no longer live like this.

Chapter 26

If Is on You to Own You

Nothing is promised to us but death. Once born, we will die. We never know when our time will come or what will happen between us. Think about this and you will realize you have no time to waste.

I choose to not have any children of mine suffer the way I did. Children should be born into the best life that we are able to afford, so that their choices are limitless. I was born in a situation where my mother and father were extremely poor. My father was a "wild" man. How many of his twenty-three children did he send to university? Not one, yet he expected us to take care of him when he was old. With his kind of thinking, how could he adequately support a woman, much less children?

This left me fighting my way through my entire educational and personal life. First, I was selling on the street, as a child in elementary school, then I was selling all the way up to my college days, when I was selling various snacks in school to buy food to put on my table. I was fortunate to receive student loans for three years out of my four to attend university. All my life I have been fighting to survive, and today I am proud of myself. I did not choose where I'd come from, but with my determination, I planned on working my way out of my poverty to a brighter future.

In a third world country, I was able to receive a Bachelor of Science in Nursing, despite the various challenges. We all have our burdens, our tests, but I worked my way through them with God as my biggest cheerleader. If I can do that, so can you. I had my family cheering me on as well. My determination was strengthened when I lived in poverty. I walked that path, I tasted it; I saw how people around me were hungry; I saw how poverty pushed young men to take up guns to get ahead, but sadly, they only lasted a few months. I used what I saw to my advantage and pledged to not go down that route. I no longer want to be a representative of poverty.

The path I chose was an honest path. It was hard, but I made it. You will go through various obstacles on the path, but when life happens, get up and go again. So here I am after the breakup of my marriage going again. I dried my tears and stopped being angry at myself because forgiving myself for being stupid will help me to forgive others.

I have learned a few tough lessons. Learning from our own mistakes can hurt so much, but it is more profound; it is embedded in our understanding of what not to do in the future. Life will never be a straight road where you can see every obstacle from afar. If it were like that, then I must say, it would be boring.

It was a hard six years of the eight years of marriage. The first two were good years because I had Nathan. I struggled through them by myself. I did not have the financial or emotional help of a husband.

I had a burning desire inside me for knowledge. I needed to know how to start managing money well. I decided to get myself educated on it. I started to read every financial book I could get my hands on. I went to the library to borrow books on the subject. I started to read and learned that knowledge is indeed power. I also started to look at the relationship between marriage and money. As I listened to the Dave Ramsey podcasts, I started to connect the dots to a better way of thinking that would help me get out of poverty.

Simply put, it's not uncommon for people who desperately want love to define love through gifts and money. I love giving gifts to others, and it's hard not to, but these habits and patterns of giving gifts recklessly should be examined.

I now know that there are four important discussions to have before marriage. I wish I had known this beforehand.

First, the topic of children should be discussed. After having Nathan, Jack declared that there would be no more children and that was it. He knew that I wanted three boys, but he was done.

Second, the topic of finances should be discussed. What are our views on this? How will we save? What will our monthly expenses look like? Should we make a weekly or monthly budget? Jack wanted me to take care of all the expenses after we were married because according to him, he had three children and I had none at the time. I blindly accepted this until the company we worked for decided that they would pay us our monthly expense stipend in one check for the household. Jack never lifted a finger, nor did he say, "Here, go buy something nice for yourself" or "Let me take you out to dinner." He never spent anything on me after the wedding, yet when he went out and about and someone asked for ten dollars, he gladly gave it to them.

The third is religion. Religion plays a major role in my life, even when I knew I was blindly making the wrong decisions. God was the source of my mother's strength through the times she had to be with my father. He was her rock. I do believe that without God in Mama's life, she would have gone permanently crazy. Here I was in a similar situation with a man who had similar characteristics to my father. You must know God to get through. Some days I cried out to God for help.

Why do we need to stay in a relationship that will break us, thinking it will get better? Looking back, when Jack pushed me in the face right in front of our son, I should have walked out of the relationship that very moment. I still remember Nathan opening his eyes so wide with fright and alarm. Tears come to my eyes when I think about that scene. Nathan should not have had to witness that. My mama was physically abused by my father, and Gina was the one who often stepped in and defended her. Even though Jack got baptized, I was naive to think that a baptism would fix his belief system. Nothing can change a man's behavior unless he is willing to change it himself.

The fourth thing to discuss is your family of origin and experiences growing up. Jack did not have a close relationship with his mother, his sisters, or his children. When his mother was alive, he did not speak highly of her. This was a warning sign I also ignored. He did not need to worry about in-laws. I later found out that his sister told him not to go to America with me because she believed the stories he told her about me. Jack's versions were half-truths. For example, he told my sister that I left him once and went to Jamaica and he did not know where I was, and he had to call my brother-in-law Ryan to find out where I was. But he failed to tell Judith why I left—he had pushed me in the face right before our two-year-old son.

My sisters and brothers and I are close. Jack was threatened by that closeness. My mother never interfered with Jack and me. She always looked at the positive. When I told her that we were getting a divorce and why, my mother cried over this for days because I had done so much for our marriage, yet this was the result. She understands now that a woman with an education can take care of herself and does not need to sit at home and take any kind of abuse from such an individual.

Mama would often say "If I could go back in my mother's womb and be reborn, I would not make this many mistakes." She stayed with my father and took the abuse. I had to explain to her that I was no longer in pain and I was a happier person since. There are no more headaches or worries that he is seeing someone else, or that Nathan and I are not getting his time. I no longer need to worry about the family decisions we need to make. I am free and single, and I can start living and loving me for me.

The opinions came from my sisters whenever I told them about a decision that I needed to make, for example, early on with the house I needed to build in Jamaica. I knew this was a solid decision. It would be a foundation to stand on. The job in the Turks and Caicos Islands was on contract, and at any time we could have been told that our services were no longer needed. Where would we go or live? When I shared this with Gina, this was her comment:

"Build yuh house, nuh mek nuh man tun yuh in a idiot. Nuh left nuh money pu dung fi him eat out. Send yuh hard earn money to Jamaica and build yuh house [Build your house. Do not allow any man to fool you. Do not leave any money in the bank for him to take. Send your money to me in Jamaica and build your house]."

This was what I did, and now I have a two-bedroom apartment rented out in Jamaica. This is my second income. It was a hard and long process, but I did it by myself without any help from Jack. If and when I am ready to move back to Jamaica, I will have a roof over my head waiting for me. Not all family members will steal your money and do what they want with it. In-laws did not interfere on my side of the family, and that was good on my part. Jack's intentions were not for us to grow together because he could only think of himself in each moment.

Marriage should not be where one person carries all the burdens. They should be shared; we carry each other's burden. Marriage should not leave you drained or make you feel enslaved. You both should shine, grow in love, and not nag, like I felt I did. During an argument, there should still be love. This love commitment should guide the relationship no matter what happens.

Breaking up with my husband has opened the windows of my mind. There are so many things I can do, but I decided to combine what I am good at with my passion. Before moving from Jamaica, I sold medical supplies and other clothing to nurses. I was good at it because I loved it. I knew what my customers wanted, and they trusted me because I was reliable. I fulfilled their needs by supplying it to them. Here in America, my plan is to do the same thing. I was at that stage once when I believed everything Jack said about his previous relationships, even when the story was not straight in my mind. I turned a blind eye. We women should question these things. My mindset of rage has been transformed now that I have insights into his views of things, and I can't be angry with any of his ex-wives.

Keeping peace is not the answer.

The answer is to live in truth.

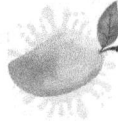

Power Thought

I now know that my legacy involves having the vulnerability to share my story in order to help others. I am using my mistakes in life as turning points. The possibilities are endless. I believe in myself now, I know I'm not crazy, I know I am motivated to create a better life than the one I came from, and I have a short time to create a retirement for myself—when I am too tired to walk. Leaving behind that old cultural mindset means that I must *be the change.*

Chapter 27

Racism in the ER

Working in the United States has made me a stronger person. The experiences I have carried for the past few years have taught me to never give up on my goals. I was a hustler in Jamaica—from selling scrunchies on the street of downtown Kingston to selling chocolate in the Northern Caribbean University. This is how I paid for my education. Life is a classroom, and the experiences we have are the lessons that fall at our desk. The daily challenges that bring us to our knees or cause us to tear up give the best education we can get. It's not what's in a textbook that you will remember as you get older and wiser, it will be those experiences. These experiences can either drain you—physically, mentally, or emotionally—or you can grow a spine and fight back.

Racism, whether some of us are aware or not, still exists. After leaving the Turks and Caicos Islands, my first assignment took me on a two-year contract to South Carolina. I have a beautiful Jamaican accent; my skin color is dark as dark chocolate. I love me now; there is nothing that I would change about this. It's part of who I am. I sometimes have patients who will go crazy over me. "Oh, I love your hair," or "I love your accent." Some even want to take pictures with me. I also have patients who have said, "Don't touch me!" Or some even went as far as calling me a nigger. Out of rebellion, I sometimes wish I were two shades darker. I know who I am and I know whose I am. I am a child of God.

One day stands out to me because it drove past the superficial tasks at hand and penetrated my soul. I took over my zone of four patients that morning and it got busier with each hour, as was expected working in the emergency room. We got to the point when each nurse had to start taking an extra patient. The hospital beds were full and as a result, patients were backed up in the ER and hall beds were lining the corridor. I recall overhearing a patient calling a family member and saying the hospital was like one of those you see on television where you have patients lining the corridors and rooms like a war zone hospital and the nurses were constantly moving. I walked away thinking how true those words were.

I loved the organized chaos, but I was tired. I looked down at my watch and felt like I could do a somersault as I only had three hours left in my long, twelve-hour shift. I would soon be able to drive home and unwind. As I bent down to adjust a hall patient's IV line, I heard the familiar sentence in my earpiece, "New patient in Room 25."

"Hey, Delpha, you got a chest-painer in your room," Sam shouted as she passed me on her way back to triage.

"I heard you in my ears a while ago."

"Hey, I got to mess with you, plus they keep coming in."

"Ah, you need to shut the doors and tell them we are out of business. Mannn." We both laughed as we continued on our separate tasks. Being a level 1 trauma center, we can't divert patients, no matter how full we are sometimes.

I grabbed my intravenous (IV) bucket and walked into my new patient's room. I smiled at the gentleman lying on a crumpled blue sheet on the bed with siderails up and head of bed elevated. I took a quick head to toe assessment to ensure that he was not in distress. I placed my IV bucket down on the table in the room as I glanced over his head and made a survey of the room to make sure my suction machine, oxygen outlet, and humidifier were still attached. Things tend to go awry quickly in the ER, and I needed to be prepared. I took a closer look at my new patient and began to calculate the things I needed to do on him. Cardiac monitor, blood pressure, oxygen saturation would need to be checked. To the left of the bed stood a petite elderly lady, wearing a loose-fitting white blouse and blue jeans, who I later learned was his wife. She wore a concerned look on her face.

I looked back at the gentleman and noticed his brown eyes had a menacing look in them. My eyes did not linger on his wrinkled face as I moved lower beside his bed to observe the rise and fall of his chest. Lowering my gaze even more, I realized that his stomach protruded. He appeared to be in his late sixties.

"Hi, my name is Delpha," I said with a smile. "I will be the nurse working with you today."

He crossed his arms over his chest.

"I am John Conerly," he belched out in an aloof tone. I turned to his wife, acknowledging her presence. "Hello, and you are?"

"I am Betsy," she said softly.

"I won't say nice to meet you because this is an unpleasant situation where I am meeting you both." I believe in taking care of the patient *and* the family members because in my mind, they are one.

His wife had a withdrawn and pensive look as she stood at his bedside. I walked over to the computer and started my charting.

"What brought you here, John—"

"How long have you been a nurse?" He interrupted me abruptly.

"I have been a nurse for over twelve years." *This should tell him I know just a little about what am doing.* He had this surprised look in his eyes when he realized that I was a registered nurse. His eyes inspected my identification badge. My qualifications were written on it.

"Well, I am a retired army doctor of twenty years," he said with unabashed pride in his voice.

I turned to him, smiled, and said, "Impressive." I could see the proudness on his face combined with a demeaning look in his eyes when he spoke to me.

Walking closer to my patient, I glanced at his wife, who was frowning, and I leaned forward on his bed. She didn't participate in our conversation. I thought I saw sadness in her eyes. Compassion welled up inside me as I thought she might be afraid of the unknown for her husband.

I tried to assist him into a hospital gown, which is when I realized how physically aggressive he was by the way that he took off his hospital shirt. He did not want me to come near him and threw the shirt at his feet, then grabbed the hospital gown from my outstretched hands. I wanted to put this man in his place, but as I looked at him, he started having difficulty with his breathing.

"Calm down," I said as I looked at the monitor. His saturation started to fall to 93 percent. "If you do not calm down, you will continue to have problems with your breathing. I am going to give you two liters of oxygen," I said, and I administered the oxygen over his scornful expression.

The only difference between both of us was the color of our skin. Should this be the cause for a barrier? I did not choose to make myself, and if that were possible, I would not change a thing. I do not want to walk around thinking I can walk on others because of the color of their skin or where they come from.

"You can leave the gown up, so I have access to your chest to put the leads on," I said with hurt in my voice.

"What did she say?" he whispered at his wife with a side glance, as if I was not there for him to ask directly.

It was a small room, and if you are good at whispering, that's fine, but I heard what he whispered to his wife. I decided to straighten up. This man would no longer see how much he was hurting me. I wanted to show him that he was not dealing with someone he could easily walk over.

"John, I know I have an accent, and sometimes I get ahead of myself, so if you do not understand me, just tell me to slow down and I will," I said, looking at the two of them directly. I repeated the request to him at a slower rate, the tears no longer in my voice. "You can leave the gown up, so I have access to your chest to put the leads on."

I started to think that this man did not like me because of the color of my skin and so I guarded myself. I did not want him to hurt me physically. I reached for the cardiac monitor leads and started to carefully stick them on his chest and attach the leads so I could see his heart rhythm.

"I see you are here for chest pain. When did it start?"

"Two days ago," he said. .."

"So, what made you come in today and not at the time you started feeling the pain?"

"It got worse."

"What were you doing when it started?"

"It woke me up."

"And did you take anything for the pain?"

"I took my nitro tablet."

"Why are you on nitro?" I asked.

"Heart attack two years ago," he abruptly stated.

I walked over to the computer desk and hooked up his EKG.

"Well, this does not show that you are having a heart attack; however, that does not mean it is not happening. As you know, there is something called a STEMI which is an ST segment elevation, and that would be positive for a myocardial infarction or a heart attack. A non-STEMI will require further tests such as cardiac enzyme bloodwork to exclude or confirm a N-STEMI. To prove that it's an N-STEMI, we will need to draw your blood, which I will explain more about later. On a scale of one to ten, how bad is it now?"

"Four," he stated under his breath.

"Were you having any shortness of breath with the chest pain?"

"Yes."

I noticed on the monitor that his SAT was 95 percent on two liters of oxygen. Despite his one- or two-word answers, I could tell he was not in distress while being inactive. I listened to his lung fields and heartbeat with my stethoscope. I wrote in his chart:

CHART ENTRY:
CRACKLES HEARD; NORMAL HEART SOUNDS AUSCULTATED. MILD PITTING EDEMA NOTED TO LOWER EXTREMITIES.

With my accent combined with his attitude, I did not want him to ask me to repeat myself or claim he did not understand what I wasn't saying. Of course, this would be beneath him. I looked in his eyes and enunciated my words:

"I will be taking your blood. We will be looking for something called a troponin. It's a cardiac enzyme, and whenever the heart muscles are damaged, it is released in the bloodstream. It takes about three to twelve hours to elevate after your symptoms start. We are also going to look at your electrolytes, such as your potassium levels, which can affect your heart."

I went on to explain everything I was going to do to him. "Which hand do you want me to stick for the IV?"

He shrugged his shoulders, glowering.
In my mind, no one would be allowed to put me down. I know what I am about and this is how I fight back—by knowing my shit.

"Hope you know what you are doing. I don't want to be stuck twice."

"Oh, I can assure you, sir, that I know what I am doing and you will not. be. stuck. twice. I popped my eyes out, with emphasis on each word." *I am going to show you who you are dealing with. I don't need to be mean to you. You have enough meanness for the two of us inside.*

This patient's overall response to me was not favorable. I tell myself that when a patient is unwelcoming that they are not in their usual environment and are now in a place where it is scary. They may be uncertain that they will recover from an illness. In this environment, they have absolutely no control. If I take away this control from an adult, my experience with that person in that moment may not be pleasant. This conduct is entirely based upon the person's character and how they handle change or stressful situations. However, this gentleman was being racist. He certainly did not respond to the doctor like that when he came into the room to talk to him. He was all pleasant and smiling.

"Hi, my name is Dr. Furgonson, and you are?"

"I am John, and this is my wife, Betsy," he said, smiling cordially.

His face was certainly not swollen like some sort of breadfruit. *Ah nice, I got to see his nasty, tobacco-stained teeth with that big smile.*

"So, what brought you here today?"

"Well, two days ago I started having pain in the center of my chest that actually woke me out of my sleep, and it reminded me of my first heart attack."

Wow, now I see that he can speak in full sentences.

I silently watched him respond to the doc with such pleasantness that I had to work extra hard to not look at him in disbelief. I glanced at his wife, who looked more or less the same as when she'd arrived. This conversation continued between John and the doctor for the next five minutes or so.

My mind began to wander. I snapped out of it when the doc took down his prescription list.

I stretched my hand out to the doctor. "Let me update them on the system, Doc."

"Thanks, Delpha. We are going to give him aspirin and at least one nitro to see if that will get rid of his chest pain. Let me know how he is doing afterward."

"Will do, Doc."

"You are in good hands with Delpha here. More than likely, you will be admitted based on your history and your current presentation. I will return when your results are back. It was nice talking to you," he said and he left the room.

As I walked out of the room to get his medication, I stopped behind the curtain separating us just long enough to bend down to pick up the paper that had just fallen out of my hands when I heard him say, "Damn niggers."

I cannot recall his wife's response to him because I had a mixture of emotions boil to the surface inside me. Everything else at that moment did not matter. As the words started to stew in my mind, I felt hurt, angry, defeated, and finally, tearful. Thank God we can no longer be bought, sold, or whipped. This hurt, but I would not let him see my response.

His cold and unwelcoming tone echoed in my ears. It hurt each time I entered his room after that, and I had to brace myself for what might come next. Several times I contemplated reporting it to my charge nurse, but with a level one adult and level two pediatric trauma center, we had a seventy-five-bed hospital area. This does not include hall beds when we are overflowing. My supervisor in charge had his hands full.

When John's blood work came back, I saw that his troponin came back positive. He was having an N-STEMI and would need to be admitted, as we suspected. He became more verbally aggressive to the point where his wife had to touch him on the shoulder and said, "Go easy."

He then turned to her and said, "I do not want a Black person to take care of me or even touch me."

"You do not have a choice. Look around, don't you see how full the hospital is? She is doing her best," said his wife.

That statement floored me. I wanted to say to him, "Meet me in the street so I can show you what I'm really made of!" In the hospital I am a professional, so of course I cannot let that side of me show. I placed my hands in my pockets and clenched my teeth and fists at the same time. I felt so powerless. He could see that he finally hit a nerve when he looked into my eyes. His eyes showed that he took great pleasure in knowing that his words affected me. I walked out of that room without saying what I really wanted to say to him.

His wife eventually left once she knew he was going to be admitted, but then he started yelling, not asking, commanding, and answering my questions in anger and in a tone that said, "How dare you even speak to me?" The tone of racism escalated with each word. At this point, I knew I had done no wrong. This was all on him.

When I walked through the open door again, my other Caucasian patient beckoned me to come over. The gentleman sympathetically apologized for this man's demeaning behavior toward me.

"I am so sorry that people like those still exist, and you need to report him."

I was very close to tearing up and could not respond to him. I walked out of the room and threw my hands in the air. "No more. I am done!"

I went to my charge nurse, which was the last thing I wanted to do as the unit was super crazy, but I had reached my limit. I said to him in my thick Jamaican accent, "I will not take care of the patient in Room 25 anymore. Find someone else to do it, man."

"Delpha, what happened?"

I turned and walked away directly to the bathroom and looked in the mirror. My eyes were red, tears pooling in them, and I sniffled. I asked the woman in the mirror, "Why am I taking this?" As my tears flowed, I thought of my four-year-old son at home, who I provided food, clothing, and shelter for. I thought about my mother who needed me. My mind began to turn. I began to yearn for something else, something bigger than this, something that I wanted to do that could be another source of income, something I could leave behind for Nathan to continue. This nursing thing was no longer a pleasure.

We were taught to never argue with a patient. It is a standard rule. If I had opened my mouth and behaved "ghetto," what would I have accomplished? He would be in the right, not because he was right but because I had handled the situation in an aggressive manner, as most people expect a Black person to do.

I left that bathroom feeling deflated yet triumphant at the same time. I was going to do what I loved. The thoughts of running my own business ran through my mind as I pulled the medication from the pyxis. My thoughts were interrupted when the charge nurse entered the room.

"Delpha, can I give you a hug?"

"No." I backed a little farther away from him in the medication room. "I am hurting too much, and if you touch me in a caring way, I will start bawling." I would not cry, but what we call it in Jamaica is "bawl" when you hurt us to the core. The pain is great, it is intense, and I knew this would take me to my knees in bawling Jamaican tears. I did not want him to hug me. Not now, not ever. When I was in my private spot, I would curl up in a ball and shed my tears.

"I need to give you a hug, Delpha." He said it with such compassion and he opened his arms and pulled me to him. In that moment I became vulnerable. I did not want to shed my tears with a "stranger" and furthermore, another Caucasian, but in that moment, he was no longer a stranger. He became a brother and a friend because he could feel my pain.

"Delpha, I had no idea that you were going through this," he said as he placed his hands on my shoulders.

I wiped my tears. "More often than you know."

"Do you know what happened? I went into the patient's room, and I spoke to him. Yes, he was being rude. But the significant part of it was that when I was walking away, the other patient called me over to tell me that for the entire evening, "that man" was being racist to you, yet you were very professional about it. You did not return the favor by being disrespectful to him. I am going to let management know about this," he said with sincerity and pain in his voice.

My charge nurse exited the medication room with his head held low. I teared up again because someone cared. I no longer felt alone in the fight against racism. I was the only Black nurse at the time working in the emergency room, but I was not the only one who felt hurt with what that patient did.

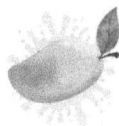

Power Statement

I look at this experience in two ways: I could choose to go ahead and classify all White people as being racist or I can say that there is both good and bad in every population. People are people no matter where they are from. If you mean to be hateful, then you will be. People can come at you from anywhere and hurt you; it's your response that counts. It's you who can invoke change.

Changes such as signs going up around the ER saying they have zero tolerance for bullying of staff members is now on display. Staff members are now aware of what being Black sometimes means to others.

Sometimes humility is the only thing we need to create awareness and change. In the moments when I felt powerless, I was empowering someone else. I was setting an example—creating an avenue for change and improvement.

I now work as a travel nurse. I have worked at several hospitals, but that one I will never forget, not because of the workload but because the camaraderie there is unmatchable to everywhere else I have worked. The experience that I gained there was priceless. I walked away with a few friends in my heart and an experience that makes me want to be an advocate for change. I am worth so much more than I knew at the time.

Chapter 28

The Feeling of Freedom

What about the parts of you that you do not like or do not want to own?

It is on you to own you.

One great psychologist told me once to look at myself in the mirror and to look at the parts of myself that I love and let these parts outshine the little parts that I don't like. He said to do this on a regular basis until I owned all of me.

Growing up, I always wanted voluptuous breasts. I wanted to wear clothing that showed them off. "I must, I must, I must increase my bust," I chanted as I looked in the mirror. I always wanted voluptuous breasts. I wanted to wear clothing that showed them off. As an adult, I still longed for the gorgeous breasts I never had as a teenager, but it was where I stood in that moment that dictated my craving for things I thought were important. From my life experience to date, I have learned to appreciate what I have in the moment. I love me for me and no longer crave a different body shape. This experience can even teach me to appreciate others around me before it is too late. Waiting until death is too late. Do it now.

If your desire to change yourself is for another person, it is the wrong reason. There will always be someone sexier than you, more beautiful than you, or more intelligent. You name it. What one might find offensive may be attractive to another. The goal is to be yourself and let your confidence shine through.

The parts that you want to change are not just physical but mental too. Do it if it will make you a better person if it builds your self-confidence. Always remember to allow God to lead in your life. Follow this principle and you will stay on track. Not only am I feeling beautiful, I also *know* that I am. I love the dark complexion of my skin. I do not use any chemicals to look lighter. I would also say that you should look at the things that you've believed about yourself that are untrue and examine them to let them go. What lies have you believed about yourself or your race or your gender, since childhood? It is time to let them go because no one can dictate your future!

I am no longer in slavery to the way my patient treated me. I will not foster the mentality of a slave either. I left that old cultural mindset behind me a long time ago. I refuse to be loud and vulgar. I can read, I have a pen and paper, and what I write tends to be louder than my voice and louder than my anger. Writing is my "inner soul voice," and I love the sound of it. I am working hard and staying focused to create a better future for my family. I want my future generations to not know the same hunger I suffered. I do not want them to have to work long hours at minimum wage to survive, living from paycheck to paycheck. I want to leave something worth leaving for Nathan for him to build on for his future generations.

I want to arrive at the point where I have diverse sources of income and can choose to live the way I want to. I recall a nurse saying to me once, "I am going to be nice to the charge nurses because they are the ones who will determine if my contract is to be renewed or not." I don't believe in sucking up to people to keep my job.

In 2020, I witnessed hospitals transition to where they had no real managers because everyone left to work as a travel nurse during the pandemic, like me. This roadrunner likes to get things done. I do not procrastinate. I always give my best to the patients, and I get the job done. I am not here to please a charge nurse or a supervisor, but I will be kind and respectful to everyone. Otherwise, I will stand up for what is right.

Black people are no longer in slavery physically, but we were not given a formula on how to stop being a mental slave or even how to handle our anger. How do we change our mindsets? It comes with practicing positive thinking and choosing the courage to improve. We live in a materialistic world, and we often think the more we have is the richer we look when sometimes our bank accounts have a zero balance, and we are in debt. The true rich man will be in brandless jeans and a T-shirt with a heavy bank account, but he walks with class and sophistication. There is a knowingness about his countenance. It shows in his eyes and by how he treats others. You know he is worth quite a lot by the inner confidence of his soul. I will not waste my money on Prada, Gucci, or whatever big brands are out there. I will spend it on what I need and not what I want until I get to where I want to be. Until then, I have a vision and a plan.

I am determined to accomplish my goals. Now, I am more of a relaxed roadrunner because I have more peace. There should be laughter in between the hardworking moments—going out with friends and family, meeting new people, and taking a chance to open up to someone you have the gut feeling to trust. Now I laugh more and go where I want to go, doing what I want to do. Now, I live up to my own expectations and not those of others.

It is up to me to own me.

This racist man I had to deal with needs to come face-to-face with his ignorance. I could not change him, nor did I seek to. I looked at myself in the mirror and questioned my actions so I could change myself, if needed, but his racism was his own.

I want to inspire you to make that change, to look at where you are going wrong and change course. No one can take you there if you are not ready to make a change.

Did I forgive the racist man for what he did? In that moment, no, I did not like him. I wanted to hurt him as much as he lashed out to hurt me. But what would be the point? What would I accomplish? Would this breakthrough the barrier of racism and change him? We are all worthy of being saved and being forgiven, just like God keeps forgiving us. I forgave him and learned from the experience. It is a memory that made me stronger. The experience showed me a new path.

Not all Black people seek violent answers to others discriminating against us. The hurt we often face in humility can be a more powerful response. As a Black nurse working in the ER, I have to prove myself even more than the others. I represent the best of the best Jamaican Black nurses. The unexpected lessons received from others are priceless. Some good came out of the experience on that terrible day with the prejudiced patient.

I recall wanting to leave Jamaica so much because I craved more, even though I didn't know what was beyond Jamaica. I just knew that I did not like how poverty felt and did not want to remain in it. I will always remember where I came from because it keeps me humble. I know who I am, I know what I want, and I know where I am going. Do I know the exact path? No, but I will learn as I travel and seek to understand, continue to better myself, and teach others how to do the same while I lead the way. Others have led the way for me, and I look to their examples. Sometimes I do fall, but I will always get back up, and I will never give up.

If you want to quit drugs, find a support group. Do not stick with someone who has the same weaknesses. Find a new group that can have a positive influence on you.

It is on you to own you.

If you are a battered wife, choose to leave. Find a way to get help and leave to build a better life, where you can thrive—a place where you can have peace of mind and are loved and respected. Learn how to love you.

It is on you to own you.

I challenge you to choose courage and take the first step toward a better you.

I started drafting this book while full of rage at my ex-husband. I was also very angry at myself for making such a life-impacting mistake by marrying the wrong person. Yet, because of finding my new love of writing, I am no longer angry. I've learned that there is nothing wrong with being separated. There is nothing wrong with being divorced. There is nothing wrong with being alone. But there is everything wrong about staying where I am not cherished, respected, valued, or loved.

I now eagerly await life's joys and challenges. I have grown. I got a divorce from someone who did not love me, nor did we have the same dream, and we were unequally yoked. The best connection we have is our beautiful son, Nathaniel. I have worked on the frontline through this pandemic at great risk to my own health. I bought a house with a beautiful, breathtaking view. I have even started to date again and am having fun. I am now more outspoken, and life does not weigh me down. I am not putting myself down, and no one else will ever try doing that again.

Can you imagine how light you might feel when you leave the stressors behind? I am no longer preoccupied with the weight on my shoulders of a problem marriage, no good insurance, or nothing saved for retirement. It's all on me to get the job done. I can just breathe and while breathing, I am blessed with a burst of energy to get me through each day.

This burst of energy helped me start my own company, Road Run-ner Medical Supplies. Get it? The me that cannot stay still is moving fast as lightning. I closed the doors to that almost as soon as I opened them. I learned that I wanted to take a different direction for my future—now that I have learned to tell my story, I am very serious about practicing my craft of writing and working on my YouTube channel instead. I now know that I'm like a diamond, with many facets to my personality and many different gifts.

My life is in the hands God gave me, and I am living with God's guidance each day. I want to listen to his voice more as he directs my path. As a single woman, I *need* to listen to his voice *first*. I also need to learn from my experiences to not repeat the pain of their effects. When the red flags go up in my head and I need to step away, I will pay atten-tion. I no longer need to feel the pressure of getting married. I have done all of that. It's time to learn more about me. God will show me who I am because he made me.

Now I want an honest, God-fearing man who takes being a leader of his home and family seriously. That is attractive to me. My father's way of managing our household was to ensure that he placed food on our table. He ensured that his children had a roof over their heads. I remember when a Category 5 hurricane hit Jamaica. Our zinc rooftop leaked as the wind blew and shook our house. He had this worried look on his face because he wanted his family to be kept safe. He saw himself as the protector. After the storm passed, he went outside and assessed the damage. He started to repair the house with a smile on his face because his family was safe. I want that kind of protector.

Because I now own the woman I am today, when others are not doing good by me [treating me right], I walk away knowing I deserve more. I have created my own happiness through loving God and doing the things I love to do with the people I love.

After five years of working in the United States of America as a registered nurse, on July 28, 2022, I was presented with my naturalization certificate. It's official. I have reached one of my goals through much determination. I am now a United States citizen. For this immigrant, this is a big achievement. The journey was a long one, but the gift is a lifelong treasure.

It's on me to own me. And things got better once I did.

I wonder what's next?

Acknowledgments

I would like to thank the following individuals for their contributions and expertise to bring my book to life:

Dr. Garland Reynolds who fact checked my ER scenes.

Thank you to Dr. Dale Okorodudu and his team at www.WhiteCoatsPublishing.com for their creative mentoring.

My Beta Readers for sharing their clarity and non-judgmental critiques: Barbara Von Der Osten, Carolette Smith, Joyce Kerr, Kelly Garrison, Neville Jones, and Tiffany Blankenship.

My hairstylists Tenisha Morrison of Crown Xtensions and Tracia Cunningham of Skindom Skin Care. I love you both as stylists and I always leave looking beautiful:

My photographer and makeup artist Tracia Cunningham of Skindom Skin Care for capturing my soul in my photos.

My graphic designers Nelton Johnson and team of Blue Ember Con-cepts Ltd, Manchester, Jamaica for being so creative.

My book project manager: Sally Hanan of Inkmeister, LLC.

A Special Thanks

Cathy Oasheim, thanks for being my friend, my coach, and my editor. You are a blessing in so many ways. Welcome to my tribe.

And Most of All

I want to thank my mother and father for helping to shape the person I am today. I love you!

If you enjoyed this book, please leave a review for it on your favorite websites. It makes all the difference for authors!

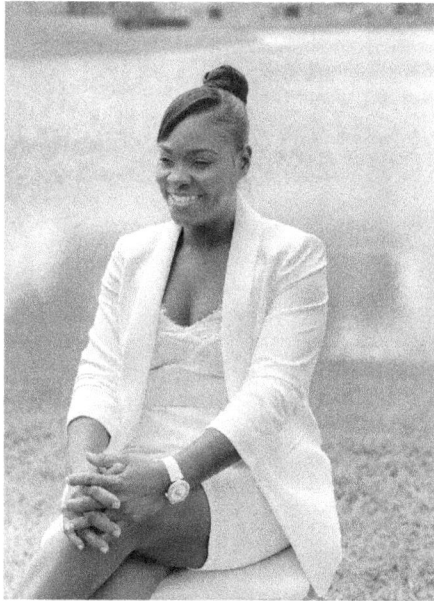

Delpha Clarke, BSN, attended the Northern Caribbean University in Mandeville Manchester, Jamaica. After four years of scraping her coins together and much hardship, she received a bachelor of science degree in nursing. She later traveled to the Turks and Caicos Islands to begin her career.

She is proud to be a newly sworn-in citizen residing in the United States and works as a traveling emergency room nurse. A love for the beach and hiking keeps her fit and motivated while she treasures her bond with her son.

Delpha's love for writing bursts with determination, faith, grit, and inspiration as she shares the depth of her soul and journey out of poverty.

delpha@delphaclarke.com
www.delphaclarke.com

If you would like to subscribe to Delpha's newsletter and get early access to future books, events, videos, and fun products, sign up via this URL: www.delphaclarke.com.

www.ingramcontent.com/pod-product-compliance
Lightning Source LLC
LaVergne TN
LVHW052023080426
835513LV00018B/2125